Nutrition for Nursing
REVIEW MODULE EDITION 6.0

Contributors

Norma Jean E. Henry, MSN/Ed, RN

Mendy McMichael, DNP, MSN

Janean Johnson, MSN, RN, CNE

Agnes DiStasi, DNP, RN, CNE

Honey C. Holman, MSN, RN

Robin A. Hertel, EdS, MSN, RN, CMSRN

Kellie L. Wilford, MSN, RN

Peggy Leehy, MSN, RN

Terri Lemon, DNP, MSN, RN

Consultants

Tracey Bousquet, BSN, RN

Penny Fauber, RN, BSN, MS, PhD

Donna Russo, RN, MSN, CCRN, CNE

Betty Daniel, MSN Nursing Education, RN

Pam DeMoss, MSN, RN

Director of content review: Kristen Lawler

Director of development: Derek Prater

Project management: Janet Hines, Nicole Burke

Coordination of content review: Norma Jean E. Henry, Mendy McMichael

Copy editing: Kelly Von Lunen, Derek Prater

Layout: Spring Lenox, Randi Hardy

Illustrations: Randi Hardy

Online media: Morgan Smith, Ron Hanson, Nicole Lobdell, Brant Stacy

Cover design: Jason Buck

Interior book design: Spring Lenox

IMPORTANT NOTICE TO THE READER

User's Guide

Welcome to the Assessment Technologies Institute® Nutrition for Nursing Review Module Edition 6.0. The mission of ATI's Content Mastery Series® Review Modules is to provide user-friendly compendiums of nursing knowledge that will:
- Help you locate important information quickly.
- Assist in your learning efforts.
- Provide exercises for applying your nursing knowledge.
- Facilitate your entry into the nursing profession as a newly licensed nurse.

This newest edition of the Review Modules has been redesigned to optimize your learning experience. We've fit more content into less space and have done so in a way that will make it even easier for you to find and understand the information you need.

ORGANIZATION

This Review Module is organized into units covering principles of nutrition, clinical nutrition, and alterations in nutrition. Chapters within these units conform to one of two organizing principles for presenting the content.
- Nursing concepts
- Nutritional considerations for specific disorders

Nursing concepts chapters begin with an overview describing the central concept and its relevance to nursing. Subordinate themes are covered in outline form to demonstrate relationships and present the information in a clear, succinct manner.

Nutritional considerations for specific disorders chapters include an overview describing nutritional needs of clients who have the given disorder. These chapters cover assessments and data collection, nutritional guidelines, nursing interventions, and complications, if applicable.

ACTIVE LEARNING SCENARIOS AND APPLICATION EXERCISES

Each chapter includes opportunities for you to test your knowledge and to practice applying that knowledge. Active Learning Scenario exercises pose a nursing scenario and then direct you to use an ATI Active Learning Template (included at the back of this book) to record the important knowledge a nurse should apply to the scenario. An example is then provided to which you can compare your completed Active Learning Template. The Application Exercises include NCLEX-style questions, such as multiple-choice and multiple-select items, providing you with opportunities to practice answering the kinds of questions you might expect to see on ATI assessments or the NCLEX. After the Application Exercises, an answer key is provided, along with rationales.

NCLEX® CONNECTIONS

To prepare for the NCLEX, it is important to understand how the content in this Review Module is connected to the NCLEX test plan. You can find information on the detailed test plan at the National Council of State Boards of Nursing's website, www.ncsbn.org. When reviewing content in this Review Module, regularly ask yourself, "How does this content fit into the test plan, and what types of questions related to this content should I expect?"

To help you in this process, we've included NCLEX Connections at the beginning of each unit and with each question in the Application Exercises Answer Keys. The NCLEX Connections at the beginning of each unit point out areas of the detailed test plan that relate to the content within that unit. The NCLEX Connections attached to the Application Exercises Answer Keys demonstrate how each exercise fits within the detailed content outline. These NCLEX Connections will help you understand how the detailed content outline is organized, starting with major client needs categories and subcategories and followed by related content areas and tasks. The major client needs categories are:
- Safe and Effective Care Environment
  - Management of Care
  - Safety and Infection Control
- Health Promotion and Maintenance
- Psychosocial Integrity
- Physiological Integrity
  - Basic Care and Comfort
  - Pharmacological and Parenteral Therapies
  - Reduction of Risk Potential
  - Physiological Adaptation

An NCLEX Connection might, for example, alert you that content within a unit is related to:
- Basic Care and Comfort
  - Nutrition and Oral Hydration
    - Manage the client who has an alteration in nutritional intake.

QSEN COMPETENCIES

As you use the Review Modules, you will note the integration of the Quality and Safety Education for Nurses (QSEN) competencies throughout the chapters. These competencies are integral components of the curriculum of many nursing programs in the United States and prepare you to provide safe, high-quality care as a newly licensed nurse. Icons appear to draw your attention to the six QSEN competencies.

Safety: The minimization of risk factors that could cause injury or harm while promoting quality care and maintaining a secure environment for clients, self, and others.

Patient-Centered Care: The provision of caring and compassionate, culturally sensitive care that addresses clients' physiological, psychological, sociological, spiritual, and cultural needs, preferences, and values.

Evidence-Based Practice: The use of current knowledge from research and other credible sources, on which to base clinical judgment and client care.

Informatics: The use of information technology as a communication and information-gathering tool that supports clinical decision-making and scientifically based nursing practice.

Quality Improvement: Care related and organizational processes that involve the development and implementation of a plan to improve health care services and better meet clients' needs.

Teamwork and Collaboration: The delivery of client care in partnership with multidisciplinary members of the health care team to achieve continuity of care and positive client outcomes.

ICONS

Icons are used throughout the Review Module to draw your attention to particular areas. Keep an eye out for these icons.

(N) This icon is used for NCLEX Connections.

(G) This icon indicates gerontological considerations, or knowledge specific to the care of older adult clients.

Qs This icon is used for content related to safety and is a QSEN competency. When you see this icon, take note of safety concerns or steps that nurses can take to ensure client safety and a safe environment.

Qpcc This icon is a QSEN competency that indicates the importance of a holistic approach to providing care.

Qebp This icon, a QSEN competency, points out the integration of research into clinical practice.

Ql This icon is a QSEN competency and highlights the use of information technology to support nursing practice.

Qqi This icon is used to focus on the QSEN competency of integrating planning processes to meet clients' needs.

Qtc This icon highlights the QSEN competency of care delivery using an interprofessional approach.

M◇ This icon appears at the top-right of pages and indicates availability of an online media supplement, such as a graphic, animation, or video. If you have an electronic copy of the Review Module, this icon will appear alongside clickable links to media supplements. If you have a hard copy version of the Review Module, visit www.atitesting.com for details on how to access these features.

FEEDBACK

ATI welcomes feedback regarding this Review Module. Please provide comments to comments@atitesting.com.

Table of Contents

NCLEX® Connections

When reviewing the following chapters, keep in mind the relevant topics and tasks of the NCLEX outline, in particular:

Client Needs: Health Promotion and Maintenance

AGING PROCESS: Provide care and education for the newborn less than 1 month old through the infant or toddler client through 2 years.

ANTE/INTRA/POSTPARTUM AND NEWBORN CARE: Provide prenatal care and education.

HEATH PROMOTION/DISEASE PREVENTION: Educate the client on actions to promote/maintain health and prevent disease.

Client Needs: Psychosocial Integrity

CULTURAL AWARENESS/CULTURAL INFLUENCES ON HEALTH: Incorporate client cultural practice and beliefs when planning and providing care.

RELIGIOUS AND SPIRITUAL INFLUENCES ON HEALTH: Evaluate whether the client's religious/spiritual needs are met.

Client Needs: Basic Care and Comfort

NUTRITION AND ORAL HYDRATION
Consider client choices regarding meeting nutritional requirements and/or maintaining dietary restrictions, including mention of specific food items.

Initiate calorie counts for clients.

Apply knowledge of mathematics to client nutrition.

UNIT 1   PRINCIPLES OF NUTRITION

CHAPTER 1   *Sources of Nutrition*

Nutrients absorbed in the diet determine, to a large degree, the health of the body. Deficiencies or excesses can contribute to a poor state of health. Essential nutrients are those that the body cannot manufacture, and the absence of essential nutrients can cause deficiency diseases.

Components of nutritive sources are carbohydrates and fiber, protein, lipids (fats), vitamins, minerals and electrolytes, and water. Carbohydrates, fats, and proteins are all energy-yielding nutrients.

DIETARY REFERENCE INTAKES

Dietary Reference Intakes (DRIs) are developed by the Institute of Medicine's Standing Committee on the Scientific Evaluation of Dietary Reference Intakes.
- The Recommended Dietary Allowance (RDA) was replaced with the DRIs in the mid-1990s.
- The DRIs are comprised of four reference values.
  ○ RDAs
  ○ Estimated Average Requirement (EAR)
  ○ Adequate Intake (AI)
  ○ Tolerable Upper Intake Level (UL)

Carbohydrates and fiber

All carbohydrates are organic compounds composed of carbon, hydrogen, and oxygen (CHO). The main function of carbohydrates is to provide energy for the body.
- The average minimum amount of carbohydrates needed to fuel the brain is 130 g/day. Median carbohydrate intake is 296 g/day among men aged 20 years and older, and 256 g/day among women in the same age range. The acceptable macronutrient distribution range for carbohydrates is 45% to 65% of calories.
- Carbohydrates provide energy for cellular work, and help to regulate protein and fat metabolism. They are essential for normal cardiac and central nervous system (CNS) functioning.

TYPES OF CARBOHYDRATES (1.1)

Carbohydrates are classified according to the number of saccharide units making up their structure.

Monosaccharides: simple carbohydrates (glucose, fructose, and galactose)

Disaccharides: simple carbohydrates (sucrose, lactose, and maltose)

Polysaccharides: complex carbohydrates (starch, fiber, and glycogen)

CONSIDERATIONS

- The liver converts fructose and galactose into glucose, which is then released in the bloodstream. This elevates blood glucose levels, which causes the release of insulin from the pancreas. With insulin production, glucose is moved out of the bloodstream into cells in order to meet energy needs.
- The body digests 95% of starch within 1 to 4 hr after ingestion. Digestion occurs mainly in the small intestine using pancreatic amylase to reduce complex carbohydrates into disaccharides.
- Glycogen is the stored carbohydrate energy source found in the liver and muscles. It is a vital source of backup energy, but is only available in limited supply.
- To maintain expected glucose levels between meals, glucose is released through the breakdown of liver glycogen.
- Digestible carbohydrates provide 4 cal/g of energy.

FIBER

Fiber is categorized as a carbohydrate.
- Dietary fiber is the substance in plant foods that is indigestible. Types are pectin, gum, cellulose, and oligosaccharides.
- Fiber is important for proper bowel elimination. It adds bulk to the feces and stimulates peristalsis to ease elimination.
- Studies show fiber helps to lower cholesterol and lessen the incidence of intestinal cancers.
- Total fiber AI is 25 g/day for women and 38 g/day for men.

1.1 Carbohydrates at a glance

	EXAMPLE (SOURCES)	FUNCTION
Monosaccharides	Glucose (corn syrup), fructose (fruits), galactose (found in milk)	Basic energy for cells
Disaccharides	Sucrose (table sugar), lactose (milk sugar), maltose (malt sugar)	Energy, aids calcium and phosphorus absorption (lactose)
Polysaccharides	Starches (grains, legumes, root vegetables), fiber (whole grains, fruits, vegetables)	Energy storage (starches), digestive aid (fiber)

Proteins

Proteins are provided by plant and animal sources. They are formed by linking amino acids in various combinations for specific use by the body.

TYPES OF PROTEINS

There are three types of proteins. Each is obtained from the diet in various ways.

Complete proteins, from animal sources and soy, contain sufficient amounts of all nine essential amino acids.

Incomplete proteins, generally from plant sources, contain all nine essential amino acids. However, one or more of the amino acids is not adequate for protein synthesis.

Complementary proteins are food sources that are incomplete proteins eaten alone, but together are equivalent to a complete protein. It is not necessary to consume complementary proteins at the same time to form a complete protein; instead, consuming a variety of complementary proteins over the course of the day is sufficient.

CONSIDERATIONS

- Proteins have many metabolic functions.
  - Tissue-building and maintenance
  - Balance of nitrogen and water
  - Backup energy
  - Support of metabolic processes
    - Nitrogen balance
    - Transportation of nutrients, other vital substances
  - Support of the immune system
- Three main factors influence the body's requirement for protein.
  - Tissue growth needs.
  - Quality of the dietary protein.
  - Added needs due to illness.
- The RDA of protein is 0.8 g/kg for healthy adults. Protein's acceptable macronutrient distribution range (AMDR) for adults is 10% to 35% of total calories.
- Underconsumption can lead to protein energy malnutrition (PEM). Kwashiorkor and marasmus are two disorders caused by extreme PEM. These serious disorders are caused by a lack of protein ingestion, or lack of protein metabolism.
- Vegan diets can lack vitamin B_{12} because it does not naturally occur in plants.
- Protein provides 4 cal/g of energy.

Lipids

- The chemical group of fats is called lipids, and they are available from many sources.
  - Dark meat
  - Poultry skin
  - Dairy foods
  - Added oils (margarine, butter, shortening, oils, lard)
- Fat is an essential nutrient for the body. It serves as a concentrated form of stored energy for the body and supplies important tissue needs.
  - Hormone production
  - Structural material for cell walls
  - Protective padding for vital organs
  - Insulation to maintain body temperature
  - Covering for nerve fibers
  - Aid in the absorption of fat-soluble vitamins

TYPES OF FATS

Fats are divided into three categories: triglycerides, phospholipids, and sterols. Triglycerides are further comprised of fatty acids, which include saturated fatty acids and unsaturated fatty acids.

Triglycerides

Triglycerides total 98% of fat in food. They combine with glycerol to supply energy to the body, allow fat-soluble vitamin transport, and form adipose tissue that protects internal organs.

- **Saturated fatty acids** are solid at room temperature, and are found primarily in animal sources.
- **Unsaturated fatty acids**, including monounsaturated and polyunsaturated fatty acids, are usually from plant sources and help reduce health risks.
  - Sources of **monounsaturated fatty acids** include olives, canola oil, avocado, peanuts and other nuts.
  - Sources of **polyunsaturated fatty acids** include corn, wheat germ, soybean, safflower, sunflower, and fish.
- **Essential fatty acids**, made from broken down fats, must be supplied by the diet. Essential fatty acids, including omega-3 and omega-6, are used to support blood clotting, blood pressure, inflammatory responses, and many other metabolic processes.

Phospholipids

Phospholipids (e.g., lecithin) are important to cell membrane structure, as well as the transport of fat-soluble substances across the cell membrane.

Sterols

Sterols (e.g., cholesterol) are found in the tissues of animals, and are not an essential nutrient because the liver is able to produce enough to meet needs.

If cholesterol is consumed in excess, it can build up in the tissues, causing congestion and increasing the risk for cardiovascular disease.

CONSIDERATIONS

- The AMDR for fats is approximately 20% to 35% of total calories. 10% or less of total calories should come from saturated fat sources).
- Cholesterol should be limited to 200 to 300 mg/day.
- A diet high in fat is linked to cardiovascular disease, hypertension, and diabetes mellitus.
  - The exception is for children under 2 years of age, who need a higher amount of fat to form brain tissue.
  - Conversely, a diet with less than 10% of fat cannot supply adequate amounts of essential fatty acids and results in a cachectic (wasting) state.
- The majority of lipid metabolism occurs after fat reaches the small intestine, where the gallbladder secretes concentrated bile and acts as an emulsifier to break fat into smaller particles. At the same time, the pancreas secretes pancreatic lipase, which breaks down fat. Intestinal cells absorb the majority of the end products of digestion, with some being excreted in the feces.
  - **Very-low-density lipoproteins (VLDL)** carry triglycerides to the cells.
  - **Low-density lipoproteins (LDL)** carry cholesterol to the tissue cells.
  - **High-density lipoproteins (HDL)** remove excess cholesterol from the cells, and transport it to the liver for disposal.
- Lipids provide 9 cal/g of energy and are the densest form of stored energy.

Vitamins

Vitamins are organic substances required for many enzymatic reactions. The main function of vitamins is to be a catalyst for metabolic functions and chemical reactions.

- There are 13 essential vitamins, each having a specialized function.
- There are two classes of vitamins.
  - **Water-soluble:** Vitamins C and B-complex
  - **Fat-soluble:** Vitamins A, D, E, and K
- Vitamins yield no usable energy for the body.

WATER-SOLUBLE VITAMINS

Vitamin C

Vitamin C (ascorbic acid) aids in tissue building and metabolic reactions (healing, collagen formation, iron absorption, immune system function).

- Vitamin C is found in citrus fruits (oranges, lemons), tomatoes, peppers, green leafy vegetables, and strawberries.
- Stress and illness, as well as cigarette smoking, increases the need for vitamin C. Cigarette smokers are advised to increase Vitamin C intake by 35 mg/day due to increased oxidative stress and metabolic turnover.
- Severe deficiency causes scurvy, a hemorrhagic disease with diffuse tissue bleeding, painful limbs/joints, weak bones, and swollen gums/loose teeth. While scurvy can be fatal, it can also be cured with moderate doses of vitamin C for several days.

B-complex vitamins

B-complex vitamins have many functions in cell metabolism. Each one has a varied duty. Many partner with other B vitamins for metabolic reactions. Most affect energy, metabolism, and neurological function. Sources for B vitamins almost always include green leafy vegetables and unprocessed or enriched grains.

Thiamin (B_1) functions as a coenzyme in energy metabolism, promotes appetite, and assists with muscle actions through its role in nerve functioning.
- Deficiency results in beriberi (ataxia, confusion, anorexia, tachycardia), headache, weight loss, and fatigue.
- Food sources are widespread in almost all plant and animal tissues, especially meats, grains, and legumes.

Riboflavin (B_2) works as a coenzyme to release energy from cells.
- Deficiency results in cheilosis (manifestations include scales and cracks on lips and in corners of the mouth), smooth/swollen red tongue (also called glossitis), and dermatitis of the ears, nose, and mouth.
- Dietary sources include milk, meats, and dark leafy vegetables.

Niacin (B_3) aids in the metabolism of fats, glucose, and alcohol.
- Deficiency causes pellagra (manifestations include sun-sensitive skin lesions, and gastrointestinal and neurological findings).
- Sources include meats, legumes, milk, whole grain and enriched breads and cereals.

Pyridoxine/Vitamin B_6 is needed for cellular function and synthesis of hemoglobin, neurotransmitters, and niacin.
- Deficiency causes macrocytic anemia and CNS disturbances.
- High intake of supplements can cause sensory neuropathy.
- Widespread food sources include meats, grains, and legumes.

Pantothenic acid is involved in the metabolism of carbohydrates, fats, and proteins as part of coenzyme A.
- Deficiency is extremely rare, but results in generalized body system failure.
- Rich sources include meats, whole grain cereals, dried peas and beans.

Biotin serves as a coenzyme used in fatty acid synthesis, amino acid metabolism, and the formation of glucose.
- Deficiency is rare, but results in neurological findings (depression, fatigue), hair loss, and scaly red rash.
- Widespread food sources include eggs, milk, and dark green vegetables.

Folate is required for hemoglobin and amino acid synthesis, new cell synthesis, and prevention of neural tube defects in utero. (Folic acid is the synthetic form.)

- Deficiency causes megaloblastic anemia, CNS disturbances, and fetal neural tube defects (spina bifida, anencephaly). It is important that all women of child-bearing age get an adequate amount of folate due to neural tube formation occurring early in gestation, often before a woman knows she is pregnant. ○EBP
- Folate occurs naturally in a variety of foods including liver, dark-green leafy vegetables, orange juice, and legumes.

Cobalamin (B₁₂) is necessary for folate activation and red blood cell maturation.

- Deficiency causes pernicious anemia and is seen mostly in strict vegans (B₁₂ is found solely in foods of animal origin), and those with the absence of intrinsic factor needed for the absorption of B₁₂.
- Sources include meat, shellfish, eggs, and dairy products.

FAT-SOLUBLE VITAMINS

- All fat-soluble vitamins have the possibility for toxicity due to their ability to be stored in the body for long periods of time.
- Absorption of fat-soluble vitamins is dependent on the body's ability to absorb dietary fat. Fat digestion can be interrupted by any number of conditions, particularly those that affect the secretion of fat-converting enzymes, and conditions of the small intestine. Clients who have cystic fibrosis, celiac disease, Crohn's disease, or intestinal bypasses are at risk for deficiencies.
- Clients who have liver disease should be careful not to take more than the daily recommendations of fat-soluble vitamins, as excess is stored in the liver and adipose tissue.

Vitamin A

Vitamin A (retinol, beta-carotene) contributes to vision health, tissue strength and growth, and embryonic development.

- Care should be taken when administered to pregnant clients as some forms have teratogenic effects on the fetus.
- Deficiency results in vision changes, xerophthalmia (dryness and hardening of the cornea), GI disturbances, and hyperkeratosis.
- Food sources include fatty fish, egg yolks, butter, cream, and dark yellow/orange fruits and vegetables (carrots, yams, apricots, squash, cantaloupe).

Vitamin D

Vitamin D assists in the absorption of calcium and phosphorus, and aids in bone mineralization.

- Sunlight enables the body to synthesize vitamin D in the skin.
- Deficiency results in bone demineralization, and extreme deficiency results in rickets. Excess consumption can cause hypercalcemia.
- Food sources include fortified milk, fatty fish, and eggs.

Vitamin E

Vitamin E is an antioxidant that helps to preserve lung and red blood cell membranes.

- Deficiency rare, but results in anemia and can cause edema and skin lesions in infants.
- Food sources include vegetable oils and certain nuts.

Vitamin K

Vitamin K assists in blood clotting and bone maintenance.

- Deficiency results in increased bleeding time.
- Used as an antidote for excess anticoagulants (warfarin).
- Vitamin K is found in carrots, eggs, and dark green vegetables (spinach, broccoli, asparagus).

1.2 Water-soluble vitamins at a glance

	MAJOR ACTIONS	MAJOR SOURCES	DEFICIENCY
Vitamin C (ascorbic acid)	Antioxidant, tissue building, iron absorption	Citrus fruits and juices, vegetables	Scurvy, decreased iron absorption, bleeding gums
Thiamin (B₁)	Muscle energy, energy metabolism	Meats, grains, legumes	Beriberi, headache, weight loss, fatigue
Riboflavin (B₂)	Assists with releasing energy from cells	Milk, meats, dark leafy vegetables	Skin eruptions, cracked lips, red swollen tongue
Niacin (B₃)	Energy and protein metabolism; cellular metabolism	Liver, nuts, legumes	Pellagra, skin lesions, GI and CNS findings, dementia
Pantothenic acid	Carbohydrate, fat, and protein metabolism	Meats, whole grain cereals, dried peas and beans.	Rare Generalized body system failure
Pyridoxine (B₆)	Cellular function, heme and neurotransmitter synthesis	Meats, grains, and legumes	Macrocytic anemia, CNS disturbances, poor growth
Folate	Synthesis of amino acids and hemoglobin, formation of fetal neural tube	Liver, green leafy vegetables, legumes	Megaloblastic anemia, CNS disturbance
Cobalamin (B₁₂)	Folate activation, red blood cell maturation	Meats, clams, oysters, eggs, dairy products	Pernicious anemia, GI findings, poor muscle coordination, paresthesia of the hands and feet

1.3 Fat-soluble vitamins at a glance

	MAJOR ACTIONS	MAJOR SOURCES	DEFICIENCY
Vitamin A	Normal vision, tissue strength, growth and immune system function	Orange/yellow fruits and vegetables, fatty fish, dairy	Reduced night vision, dry/thick corneas, mucosa changes
Vitamin D	Maintain serum calcium and phosphorus, aid in bone development	Fish, fortified dairy products, egg yolks, sunlight	Low serum calcium, fragile bones, rickets, osteomalacia in adults
Vitamin E	Protects vitamin A from oxidation	Vegetable oils, grains, nuts, dark green vegetables	Anemia, edema and skin lesions in infants
Vitamin K	Essential for prothrombin synthesis, aids in bone metabolism	Green leafy vegetables, eggs	Increased bleeding times

Minerals and electrolytes

Minerals are available in an abundance of food sources and are used at every cellular level for metabolic exchanges. Minerals are divided into major and trace.

MAJOR MINERALS

Major minerals occur in larger amounts (more than 5 g) in the body, and 100 mg or more is required through dietary sources each day. The seven major minerals are calcium, phosphorus, sodium, potassium, magnesium, chloride, and sulfur.

Electrolytes

Electrolytes are electrically charged minerals that cause physiological reactions that maintain homeostasis. Major minerals include sodium, potassium, and chloride.

Sodium (Na)

MAJOR ACTIONS: Maintains fluid volume, allows muscle contractions, contributes to nerve impulses

MAJOR SOURCES: Table salt, added salts, processed foods

FINDINGS OF DEFICIENCY: Muscle cramping, memory loss, anorexia

FINDINGS OF EXCESS: Fluid retention, hypertension, disorientation

NURSING CONSIDERATIONS: Monitor level of consciousness, edema, and blood pressure.

Potassium (K)

MAJOR ACTIONS: Maintains fluid volume inside cells, muscle action

MAJOR SOURCES: Oranges, dried fruits, tomatoes, avocados, dried peas, meats, broccoli, bananas, dairy products, meats, whole grains

FINDINGS OF DEFICIENCY: Dysrhythmias, muscle cramps, confusion

FINDINGS OF EXCESS: Dysrhythmia, muscle weakness, irritability, confusion, numbness in extremities

NURSING CONSIDERATIONS: Monitor cardiac status and ECG. PO tabs irritate the GI system. Give with meals.

Chloride (Cl)

MAJOR ACTIONS: Assists with intracellular and extracellular fluid balance, aids digestion

MAJOR SOURCES: Table salt

FINDINGS OF DEFICIENCY: Rare; muscle cramps, anorexia

FINDINGS OF EXCESS: Vomiting

NURSING CONSIDERATIONS: Monitor sodium levels.

Calcium (Ca)

MAJOR ACTIONS: Bones/teeth formation, blood pressure, blood clotting, nerve transmission

MAJOR SOURCES: Dairy, broccoli, kale, grains, egg yolks

FINDINGS OF DEFICIENCY: Tetany, positive Chvostek's and Trousseau's signs, ECG changes, osteoporosis in adults, poor growth in children

FINDINGS OF EXCESS: Constipation, renal stones, lethargy, depressed deep-tendon reflexes

NURSING CONSIDERATIONS: Monitor ECG and respiratory status. Give PO tabs with vitamin D.

Magnesium (Mg)

MAJOR ACTIONS: Bone formation, catalyst for many enzyme reactions, nerve/muscle function, smooth muscle relaxation

MAJOR SOURCES: Green leafy vegetables, nuts, whole grains, tuna, halibut, chocolate

FINDINGS OF DEFICIENCY: Weakness, dysrhythmias, vertigo, convulsions, increased blood pressure, anorexia

FINDINGS OF EXCESS: Diarrhea, nausea, muscle weakness, hypotension, bradycardia, lethargy

NURSING CONSIDERATIONS: Seizure precautions, monitor level of consciousness and vital signs Qs

Phosphorus (P)

MAJOR ACTIONS: Energy transfer of RNA/DNA, acid-base balance, bone and teeth formation

MAJOR SOURCES: Dairy, peas, meat, eggs, legumes

FINDINGS OF DEFICIENCY: Unknown

FINDINGS OF EXCESS: Decreased serum calcium levels

NURSING CONSIDERATIONS: Evaluate the use of antacids (note type) and the use of alcohol (alcohol impairs absorption).

Sulfur (S)

MAJOR ACTIONS: A component of vitamin structure, by-product of protein metabolism

MAJOR SOURCES: Proteins

FINDINGS OF DEFICIENCY: Only seen in severe protein malnourishment

FINDINGS OF EXCESS: Toxicity does not result in any health issues

NURSING CONSIDERATIONS: Sulfur levels are not usually monitored.

TRACE MINERALS

Trace minerals, also called micronutrients, are required by the body in amounts of less than 5 g, and 20 mg or less is required through dietary sources each day. The nine trace elements are iron, iodine, zinc, copper, manganese, chromium, selenium, molybdenum, and fluoride.

Iodine

Iodine is used for synthesis of thyroxine, the thyroid hormone that helps regulate metabolism. Iodine is taken up by the thyroid. When iodine is lacking, the thyroid gland enlarges, creating a goiter.

- Grown food sources vary widely and are dependent on the iodine content of the soil in which they were grown.
- Seafood provides a good amount of iodine. Table salt in the U.S. is fortified with iodine, so deficiencies are not as prevalent.
- The RDA is 150 mcg for adults.

Iron

Iron is responsible for oxygen distribution to hemoglobin and myoglobin.

- The body recycles unused iron from dying red blood cells and stores it for later use.
- Iron in food consists of two forms; heme iron found in meat, fish and poultry and nonheme iron found in grains, legumes, and vegetables.
- Iron supplements can cause constipation, nausea, vomiting, diarrhea, and teeth discoloration (liquid form). They can be taken with food to avert gastrointestinal symptoms, and nurses should encourage fresh fruits, vegetables, and a high-fiber diet.
- Supplements that are unneeded can become toxic.

- Intramuscular injections are caustic to tissues and must be administered by Z-track method.
- Vitamin C increases the absorption of iron.
- Females during the menstruating years, older infants and toddlers and pregnant women are at risk for iron deficiency anemia.

Fluoride

Fluoride forms a bond with calcium and thus accumulates in calcified body tissue (bones and teeth). Water with added fluoride protects against dental cavities.

Water

Water is the most basic of nutrients. The body can maintain itself for several weeks on its food stores of energy, but it cannot survive without water/hydration for more than a few days. Water makes up the largest portion of our total body weight and is crucial for all fluid and cellular functions.

- Fluid balance is essential for optimum health and bodily function.
- The balance of fluid is a dynamic process regulated by the release of hormones.
- To maintain a balance between intake and output, intake should approximate output. Healthy adults lose approximately 1000 mL of water daily through insensible losses (respirations, skin, fecal), and to get rid of metabolic wastes needs to excrete at least 500 mL of urine daily. Therefore, the minimum daily amount of water intake needed is 1,500 mL.
- Under normal conditions, the AI for adult fluid intake is 3 L/day for men and 2.2L/day for women.
- Additional hydration can be required for athletes, persons with fever/illness (vomiting, diarrhea), and those in hot climate conditions.
- Young children and older adults dehydrate more rapidly.
- Clients who cannot hold down fluid or must withhold fluids in preparation for a procedure may be hydrated with intravenous fluids.
- Water leaves the body via the kidneys, skin, lungs, and feces. The greatest elimination is through the kidneys. Other loss factors to be considered include bleeding, vomiting, and rapid respirations. Persistent vomiting can quickly dehydrate a person.
- A balanced input/output ratio is almost 1:1. Nurses should consider the health status and individual needs of the client.
- Assessment for proper hydration should include skin turgor, mental status, orthostatic blood pressures, urine output and concentration, and moistness of mucous membranes.
- Thirst is a late sign of the need for hydration, especially in older adults.
- Some individuals can have an aversion to drinking water, and should be encouraged to explore other options (fresh fruits, fruit juices, flavored gelatin, frozen treats, soups).
- Caffeinated drinks have a diuretic effect and should not be substituted for other fluids.

Application Exercises

1. A nurse is educating a client who is taking iron supplements about foods which aid in iron absorption. Which of the following foods is the best choice for the client to make?

   A. 1 baked potato

   B. ½ cup orange juice

   C. ½ cup low-fat milk

   D. 2 cups boiled green beans

2. A nurse is discussing foods that are high in vitamin D with a client who is unable to be out in the sunlight. Which of the following should be included in the teaching?

   A. 1 cup steamed long-grain brown rice

   B. 6 medium raw strawberries

   C. ½ cup boiled Brussels sprouts

   D. 2 large, poached eggs

3. A nurse is caring for a client who is prescribed warfarin. The nurse should teach the client that which of the following vitamins can interfere with this medication?

   A. Vitamin A

   B. Vitamin D

   C. Vitamin E

   D. Vitamin K

4. A nurse is conducting a nutritional class on minerals and electrolytes. The nurse should include that ½ cup of which of the following foods is the best source of magnesium?

   A. Whole almonds

   B. Chopped tomatoes

   C. Raw spinach

   D. Low-fat vanilla yogurt

5. A nurse is discussing health problems associated with nutrient deficiencies with a group of adolescents. The nurse should include that which of the following conditions is associated with a deficiency of vitamin C?

   A. Dysrhythmias

   B. Scurvy

   C. Pernicious anemia

   D. Megaloblastic anemia

PRACTICE Active Learning Scenario

A school nurse is conducting a nutritional class for a group of athletes. Use the ATI Active Learning Template: Basic Concept to complete this item.

RELATED CONTENT

Describe three types of protein.

Describe three main factors influencing the body's requirement for protein.

Application Exercises Key

1. A. One baked potato has 20 mg of vitamin C, and is not the best food choice for the client to make.

   B. **CORRECT:** Vitamin C aids in the absorption of iron, and ½ cup orange juice has 62 mg of vitamin C. This is the best food choice for the client to make.

   C. ½ cup low-fat milk has 1.2 mg of vitamin C, and is not the best food choice for the client to make.

   D. Two cups green beans has 24 mg of vitamin C, and is not the best food choice for the client to make.

   Ⓝ *NCLEX® Connection: Basic Care and Comfort, Nutrition and Oral Hydration*

2. A. Long-grain brown rice does not contain vitamin D.

   B. Strawberries do not contain vitamin D.

   C. Brussels sprouts do not contain vitamin D.

   D. **CORRECT:** The nurse should include eggs as a food that is high in vitamin D.

   Ⓝ *NCLEX® Connection: Basic Care and Comfort, Nutrition and Oral Hydration*

3. A. Vitamin A does not interfere with warfarin

   B. Vitamin D does not interfere with warfarin.

   C. Vitamin E does not interfere with warfarin.

   D. **CORRECT:** Vitamin K assists in blood clotting, is used as an antidote for excess anticoagulants, and can interfere with warfarin. The nurse should instruct the client to avoid increasing sources of vitamin K through supplements or in the diet.

   Ⓝ *NCLEX® Connection: Basic Care and Comfort, Nutrition and Oral Hydration*

4. A. **CORRECT:** ½ cup whole almonds is the best source because it has 193 mg of magnesium.

   B. ½ cup chopped red tomatoes is not the best source because it has 10 mg of magnesium.

   C. ½ cup raw spinach is not the best source because it has 12 mg of magnesium.

   D. ½ cup low-fat vanilla yogurt is not the best source because it has 20 mg of magnesium.

   Ⓝ *NCLEX® Connection: Physiological Adaptation, Fluid and Electrolyte Imbalances*

5. A. Dysrhythmias are associated with a potassium deficiency.

   B. **CORRECT:** Scurvy is associated with a vitamin C deficiency.

   C. Pernicious anemia is associated a deficiency of vitamin B_{12}.

   D. Megaloblastic anemia is associated with a deficiency of folate.

   Ⓝ *NCLEX® Connection: Physiological Adaptation, Illness Management*

PRACTICE Answer

Using the ATI Active Learning Template: Basic Concept

RELATED CONTENT

- Types of protein
  - Complete proteins, from animal sources and soy, contain sufficient amounts of all nine essential amino acids.
  - Incomplete proteins, generally from plants sources, contain all nine essential amino acids. However, one or more of the amino acids is not adequate for protein synthesis.
  - Complementary proteins are those food sources that are incomplete proteins eaten alone, but together are equivalent to a complete protein. It is not necessary to consume complementary proteins at the same time to form a complete protein; instead, consuming a variety of complementary proteins over the course of the day is sufficient.
- Main factors influencing the body's requirement for protein
  - Tissue growth needs
  - Quality of the dietary protein
  - Added needs due to illness

Ⓝ *NCLEX® Connection: Health Promotion and Maintenance, Health Promotion/Disease Prevention*

UNIT 1   PRINCIPLES OF NUTRITION

CHAPTER 2 *Ingestion, Digestion, Absorption, and Metabolism*

Ingestion is the process of consuming food by the mouth, and moving it through the digestive system. Digestion is a systemic process that includes the breakdown and absorption of nutrients.

Absorption occurs as components of nutrients pass through the digestive system into the bloodstream and lymphatic system. Medication absorption can be affected by food intake. It is important for nurses to be aware of food and medication absorption. Nurses should assess liver and kidney functioning to determine adequacy prior to medication administration.

Metabolism is the sum of all chemical processes that occur on a cellular level to maintain homeostasis. Nutrients from food must enter a cell in order for metabolism to occur. Metabolism is comprised of two processes: catabolism (the breaking down of substances with the resultant release of energy) and anabolism (the use of energy to build or repair substances).

Energy nutrients are metabolized to provide carbon dioxide, water, and adenosine triphosphate (ATP). Excess energy nutrients are stored; glucose is converted to glycogen and stored in the liver and muscle tissue; surplus glucose is converted to fat; glycerol and fatty acids are reassembled into triglycerides and stored in adipose tissue; and amino acids make body proteins. The liver removes excess amino acids and uses the residue to form glucose or store it as fat. Body cells first use available ATP for growth and repair, then use glycogen and stored fat.

METABOLIC RATE

Metabolic rate refers to the speed at which food energy is burned.

- **Basal metabolic rate (BMR)**, also called basal energy expenditure (BEE), refers to the amount of energy used in 24 hr for involuntary activities of the body, such as maintaining body temperature, heartbeat, circulation, and respirations. This rate is determined while at rest, and following a 12-hr fast.
- **Resting metabolic rate (RMR)**, also called resting energy expenditure (REE), refers to the calories needed for involuntary activities of the body at rest. This rate does not consider the 12-hr fast criteria.
- BMR is affected by lean body mass and hormones. Body surface area, age, and gender are also factors that contribute to BMR.
- In general, men have a higher metabolic rate than women due to their higher amount of body muscle and decreased amount of fat.
- Thyroid function tests can be used as an indirect measure of BMR.
- Acute stress causes an increase in metabolism, blood glucose levels, and protein catabolism.
  - A major nutritional concern during acute stress is protein deficiency as stress hormones break down protein at a very rapid rate.
  - Protein deficiency increases the risk of complications from severe trauma or critical illness (skin breakdown, delayed wound healing, infections, organ failure, ulcers, impaired medication tolerance).
  - Protein requirements may be increased to more than 2 g/kg of body weight, or up to 25% of total calories, depending on the client's age and prior nutritional status.
- Any catabolic illness (surgery, extensive burns) increases the body's requirement for calories to meet the demands of an increased BMR.
- Disease and sepsis also increase metabolic demands and can lead to starvation/death.

FACTORS AFFECTING METABOLIC RATE

INCREASE BMR
- Lean, muscular body build
- Exposure to extreme cold
- Prolonged stress
- Rapid growth periods (infancy, puberty)
- Pregnancy
- Lactation
- Physical conditioning

DECREASE BMR
- Short, overweight body build
- Starvation/malnutrition
- Age older than 60 years

Conditions

INCREASE METABOLISM
- Fever
- Involuntary muscle tremors (e.g., shivering, Parkinson's)
- Hyperthyroidism
- Cancer
- Cardiac failure
- Diabetes mellitus
- Burns
- Surgery/wound healing
- HIV/AIDS

DECREASE METABOLISM: Hypothyroidism

Medications

INCREASE BMR
- Prednisone
- Epinephrine
- Levothyroxine
- Ephedrine sulfate

DECREASE BMR: Amitriptyline

NITROGEN BALANCE

Nitrogen balance refers to the difference between the daily intake and excretion of nitrogen. It is also an indicator of tissue integrity. A healthy adult experiencing a stable weight is in nitrogen equilibrium, also known as neutral nitrogen balance.

Positive nitrogen balance indicates that the intake of nitrogen exceeds excretion. Specifically, the body builds more tissue than it breaks down. This normally occurs during periods of growth: infancy, childhood, adolescence, pregnancy, and lactation.

Negative nitrogen balance indicates that the excretion of nitrogen exceeds intake. The individual is receiving insufficient protein, and the body is breaking down more tissue than it is building, as seen during periods of illness, trauma, aging, and malnutrition.

ASSESSMENT/DATA COLLECTION

- Weight and history of recent weight patterns
- Medical history for diseases that affect metabolism and nitrogen balance
- Extent of traumatic injuries, as appropriate
- Fluid and electrolyte status
- Laboratory values: albumin, transferrin, glucose, and creatinine
- Clinical signs of malnutrition: pitting edema, hair loss, and wasted appearance
- Medication side effects that can affect nutrition
- Usual 24-hr dietary intake
- Use of nutritional supplements, herbal supplements, vitamins, and minerals
- Use of alcohol, caffeine, and nicotine

NURSING INTERVENTIONS

- Monitor food intake.
- Monitor fluid intake and output.
- Use patient-centered approach to address disease-specific problems with ingestion, digestion, or medication regime. ℚpcc
- Collaborate with nutritionist.
- Provide adequate calories and high-quality protein.

STRATEGIES TO INCREASE PROTEIN, CALORIC CONTENT
- Add skim milk powder to milk (double-strength milk).
- Use whole milk instead of water in recipes.
- Add cheese, peanut butter, chopped hard-boiled eggs, or yogurt to foods.
- Dip meats in eggs or milk and coat with bread crumbs before cooking.
- Nuts and dried beans are significant sources of protein. These are good alternatives for a dairy allergy or lactose intolerance.

Application Exercises

1. A nurse is caring for a client who has hypothyroidism. Which of the following is associated with this disorder?

   A. Decreased metabolic demand

   B. Weight loss

   C. Increased heart rate

   D. Diarrhea

2. A nurse is reviewing prescribed medications for a newly admitted client. Which of the following medications decreases the body's rate of metabolism?

   A. Prednisone

   B. Levothyroxine

   C. Amitriptyline

   D. Epinephrine

3. A charge nurse is conducting a nutritional class for a group of newly licensed nurses regarding basal metabolic rate (BMR). The charge nurse should inform the class that which of the following factors increases BMR? (Select all that apply.)

   A. Lactation

   B. Prolonged stress

   C. Malnutrition

   D. Puberty

   E. Age older than 60 years

4. A school nurse is teaching a high school health class about the possible causes of a negative nitrogen balance. Which of the following causes should the nurse include in the teaching? (Select all that apply.)

   A. Illness

   B. Malnutrition

   C. Adolescence

   D. Trauma

   E. Pregnancy

PRACTICE Active Learning Scenario

A nurse is conducting a nutritional program for a group of newly licensed nurses regarding ingestion, digestion, absorption, and metabolism. Use the ATI Active Learning Template: Basic Concept to complete this item.

RELATED CONTENT: Identify three components of absorption.

Application Exercises Key

1. A. **CORRECT:** A decreased metabolic demand is associated with hypothyroidism.

   B. Weight gain, not weight loss, is associated with hypothyroidism.

   C. Bradycardia, not tachycardia, is associated with hypothyroidism.

   D. Constipation, not diarrhea, is associated with hypothyroidism.

   Ⓝ *NCLEX® Connection: Health Promotion and Maintenance, Aging Process*

2. A. Prednisone is a glucocorticoid used for suppressing the immune system and inflammation. This medication increases the body's rate of metabolism.

   B. Levothyroxine is used for the treatment of hypothyroidism and increases the body's rate of metabolism.

   C. **CORRECT:** Amitriptyline is tricyclic antidepressant used for treating depression and decreases the body's rate of metabolism.

   D. Epinephrine is used to treat acute asthma attacks and anaphylaxis, and increases the body's rate of metabolism.

   Ⓝ *NCLEX® Connection: Physiological Adaptation, Illness Management*

3. A. **CORRECT:** The charge nurse should include in the teaching that lactation increases BMR.

   B. **CORRECT:** The charge nurse should include in the teaching that prolonged stress increases BMR.

   C. The nurse should include in the teaching that malnutrition decreases BMR.

   D. **CORRECT:** The nurse should include in the teaching that puberty increases BMR.

   E. The nurse should include in the teaching that being over 60 years of age decreases BMR.

   Ⓝ *NCLEX® Connection: Health Promotion and Maintenance, Aging Process*

4. A. **CORRECT:** Illness is a possible cause of negative nitrogen balance.

   B. **CORRECT:** Malnutrition is a possible cause of negative nitrogen balance.

   C. Adolescence is a possible cause of positive nitrogen balance.

   D. **CORRECT:** Trauma is a possible cause of negative nitrogen balance.

   E. Pregnancy is a possible cause of positive nitrogen balance.

   Ⓝ *NCLEX® Connection: Physiological Adaptation, Illness Management*

PRACTICE Answer

Using the ATI Active Learning Template: Basic Concept

RELATED CONTENT

- Absorption occurs as components of nutrients pass through the digestive system into the bloodstream and lymphatic system.
- Medication absorption can be affected by food intake. It is important for nurses to be aware of food and medication absorption.
- Nurses should assess liver and kidney functioning to determine adequacy prior to medication administration.

Ⓝ *NCLEX® Connection: Health Promotion and Maintenance, Aging Process*

CHAPTER 3 *Nutrition Assessment/ Data Collection*

Nurses play a key role in assessing the nutritional needs of clients. Nurses monitor and intervene with clients requiring acute and chronic nutritional care. Nurses should consider and incorporate the family's nutritional habits into a client's individual plan of care. Nurses should take an active role in assessing and teaching community groups regarding nutrition.

A collaborative, interprofessional approach provides the best outcomes for the client. Providers and nurses collect physical assessment data. Registered dietitians complete comprehensive nutritional assessments. Nurses monitor and evaluate interventions provided to clients. Q꜀

A client's physical appearance can be deceiving. A client who has a healthy weight and appearance can be malnourished. Cultural, social, and physical norms must be part of a client's assessment. Even with adequate client education, personal preferences can be an overriding factor to successful nutritional balance.

DIET HISTORY

A diet history is an assessment of usual foods, fluids, and supplements. Components include the following.
- Time, type, and amount of food eaten for breakfast, lunch, dinner, and snacks
- Time, type, and amount of fluids consumed throughout the day, including water, health drinks, coffee/tea, carbonated beverages, and beverages with caffeine
- Type, amount, and frequency of "special foods" (celebration foods, movie foods)
- Typical preparation of foods and fluids (coffee with sugar, fried foods)
- Number of meals eaten away from home (at work or school)
- Type of preferred or prescribed diet (ovo–lacto vegetarian, 2 g sodium/low–fat diet)
- Foods avoided due to allergy or preference
- Frequency and dose/amount of medications or nutritional supplements taken daily
- Satisfaction with diet over a specified time frame (last 3 months, 1 year)

TOOLS TO DETERMINE NUTRITIONAL STATUS

A physical assessment is performed by the provider or nurse to identify indicators of inadequate nutrition. However, other diseases, or conditions can cause these clinical findings.

MANIFESTATIONS
- Hair that is dry or brittle, or skin that has dry patches
- Poor wound healing or sores
- Lack of subcutaneous fat or muscle wasting
- Irregular cardiovascular measurements (heart rate and rhythm, blood pressure)
- Enlarged spleen or liver
- General weakness or impaired coordination

ANTHROPOMETRIC TOOLS

Weight
- Weigh at the same time of day wearing similar clothing to ensure accurate weight readings.
- Daily fluctuations generally are indicative of water weight changes.
- Percentage weight change calculation (weight change over a specified time):

$$\% \text{ weight change} = \frac{(\text{usual weight - present weight})}{\text{usual weight}} \times 100$$

  - Greater than 2% in 1 week indicates a significant weight loss.
  - Greater than 7.5% in 3 months indicates a significant weight loss.
- "Ideal" body weight based on height (plus or minus 10% depending on frame size).
  - **MALES:** 48 kg (106 lb) for the first 152 cm (5 ft) of height, and 2.7 kg (6 lb) for each additional 2.5 cm (1 in).
  - **FEMALES:** 45 kg (100 lb) for the first 152 cm (5 ft) of height, and 2.3 kg (5 lb) for each additional 2.5 cm (1 in).

Height
- Measure on a vertical, flat surface. Ask the client to remove shoes and head coverings and stand straight with heels together looking straight ahead.
- Obtain a recumbent measurement (lying on a firm, flat surface) for infants and young children.

Body mass index (BMI)
- Healthy weight is indicated by a BMI of 18.5 to 24.9.
- Overweight is defined as an increased body weight in relation to height. It is indicated by a BMI of 25 to 29.9.
- Obesity is an excess amount of body fat. It indicated by a BMI greater than or equal to 30.

$$\text{BMI} = \text{weight (kg)} \div \text{height (m}^2)$$

CLINICAL VALUES

Fluid intake and output (I&O)
- Adults: 2,000 to 3,000 mL (2 to 3 L) per day
- Total average output: 1,750 to 3,000 mL/day

Protein levels are measured by serum albumin levels. Many non-nutritional factors (injury or kidney disease), interfere with this measure for protein malnutrition.

Prealbumin (thyroxine-binding protein) is a sensitive measure used to assess critically ill clients who are at risk for malnutrition. This test reflects acute changes rather than gradual changes. However, it is more expensive and often unavailable. This is not part of routine assessment.
- Prealbumin levels can decrease with an inflammatory process resulting in an inaccurate measurement.
- Prealbumin levels are used to measure effectiveness of total parenteral nutrition.

3.1 Clinical laboratory tests

	EXPECTED REFERENCE RANGE	MODERATE DEPLETION
Albumin	3.5 to 5.0 g/dL	2.4 to 2.9 g/dL
Prealbumin	15 to 36 mg/dL	less than 10.7 mg/dL

Nitrogen balance refers to the relationship between protein breakdown (catabolism) and protein synthesis (anabolism).
- To measure nitrogen balance
  - Record protein intake (g) over 24 hr and divide by 6.25.
  - Record nitrogen excretion in urine over 24 hr and add 4 g.
  - Subtract nitrogen output from nitrogen intake.
  - 24 hr protein intake ÷ 6.25 = nitrogen intake (g)
  - 24 hr urinary urea nitrogen + 4 g = total nitrogen output

  Nitrogen intake - total nitrogen output = nitrogen balance

- A neutral nitrogen balance indicates adequate nutritional intake
- A positive nitrogen balance indicates protein synthesis is greater than protein breakdown as during growth, pregnancy, or during recovery.
- A negative nitrogen balance indicates protein is used at a greater rate than it is synthesized as in starvation or a catabolic state following injury or disease.

RISK FACTORS FOR INADEQUATE NUTRITION

BIOPHYSICAL FACTORS
- Medical disease/conditions/treatment (hypertension, HIV/AIDS, surgery)
- Genetic predisposition (lactose intolerance, osteoporosis)
- Age

PSYCHOLOGICAL FACTORS
- Mental illness (clinical depression)
- Excessive stress
- Negative self-concept
- Use of comfort foods

SOCIOECONOMIC FACTORS
- Poverty
- Alcohol and other substance use disorders
- Fad or "special" diets
- Food preferences: cultural, ethnic, or religious

EFFECT OF RISK FACTORS ON NUTRITIONAL STATUS

The following are examples of how risk factors can affect nutritional status.
- A client has edema and requires treatment with a diuretic and low-sodium diet. Diuretics can cause sodium and potassium imbalances. A low-sodium diet can be unappetizing and cause inadequate consumption.
- Osteoporosis has many modifiable risk factors (calcium and vitamin D intake, inactive lifestyle, cigarette smoking, alcohol intake). Altering these risk factors can affect nutritional status in a positive manner.
- Poor self-concept can cause a client to avoid needed foods and nutrients, or to overeat.

Application Exercises

1. A nurse in a nutritional clinic is calculating body mass index (BMI) for several clients. The nurse should recognize which of the following client BMIs as overweight?

   A. BMI of 24

   B. BMI of 30

   C. BMI of 27

   D. BMI of 32

2. A nurse on an orthopedic unit is reviewing data for a client who sustained trauma in a motor-vehicle crash. Which of the following values indicates the client is in a catabolic state (using protein faster than protein is being synthesized)?

   A. Serum albumin 3.5 g/dL.

   B. Negative nitrogen balance.

   C. BMI of 18.5.

   D. Serum prealbumin 12 mg/dL.

3. A nurse is performing a nutritional assessment on a client. Which of the following clinical findings are suggestive of malnutrition? (Select all that apply.)

   A. Poor wound healing

   B. Dry hair

   C. Blood pressure 130/80 mm Hg

   D. Weak hand grips

   E. Impaired coordination

4. A nurse is teaching a group of women about risk factors for developing osteoporosis. Which of the following risk factors should the nurse include? (Select all that apply.)

   A. Inactivity

   B. Family history

   C. Obesity

   D. Hyperlipidemia

   E. Cigarette smoking

PRACTICE Active Learning Scenario

A community health nurse is conducting a dietary assessment for a client. Use the ATI Active Learning Template: Basic Concept to complete this item.

UNDERLYING PRINCIPLES: Describe four components of a diet history.

Application Exercises Key

1. A. A healthy weight is indicated by a BMI of 18.5 to 24.9.

    B. Obesity is an excess amount of body fat indicated by a BMI greater than or equal to 30.

    C. **CORRECT:** Overweight is defined as an increased body weight in relation to height, indicated by a BMI of 25 to 29.9.

    D. Obesity is an excess amount of body fat indicated by a BMI greater than or equal to 30.

    Ⓝ *NCLEX® Connection: Basic Care and Comfort, Nutrition and Oral Hydration*

2. A. Serum albumin levels reflect slow changes in serum protein levels, not acute serum protein changes. A serum albumin of 3.5 g/dL or 4.5 g/dL is within the expected reference range.

    B. **CORRECT:** A negative nitrogen balance indicates protein is used at a greater rate than it is synthesized as in starvation or a catabolic state following injury or disease.

    C. A BMI of 18.5 indicates an ideal body weight.

    D. A serum prealbumin of 15 mg/dL is within the expected reference range.

    Ⓝ *NCLEX® Connection: Reduction of Risk Potential, Laboratory Values*

3. A. **CORRECT:** Poor wound healing describes changes reflective of malnutrition.

    B. **CORRECT:** Dry hair describes changes reflective of malnutrition.

    C. A blood pressure value of 130/80 mm Hg is an expected cardiovascular finding and is not associated with malnutrition.

    D. **CORRECT:** Weak hand grips describe changes reflective of malnutrition.

    E. **CORRECT:** Impaired coordination describes changes reflective of malnutrition.

    Ⓝ *NCLEX® Connection: Basic Care and Comfort, Nutrition and Oral Hydration*

4. A. **CORRECT:** There is an increased risk for osteoporosis due to inactivity. Weight-bearing exercises is a primary prevention measure.

    B. **CORRECT:** A family history of osteoporosis is a risk factor.

    C. Weight loss can cause a decreased intake of dietary calcium and vitamin D, leading to the development of osteoporosis.

    D. Hyperlipidemia is not a risk factor for the development of osteoporosis in women.

    E. **CORRECT:** Cigarette smoking can increase the incidence of osteoporosis.

    Ⓝ *NCLEX® Connection: Health Promotion and Maintenance, Health Promotion/Disease Prevention*

PRACTICE Answer

Using the ATI Active Learning Template: Basic Concept

UNDERLYING PRINCIPLES: A diet history is an assessment of usual foods, fluids, and supplements.

- Time, type, and amount of food eaten for breakfast, lunch, dinner, and snacks.
- Time, type, and amount of fluids consumed throughout the day including water, health drinks, coffee/tea, carbonated beverages, and beverages with caffeine.

- Type, amount, and frequency of "special foods" (celebration foods, movie foods).
- Typical preparation of foods and fluids (coffee with sugar, fried foods).
- Number of meals eaten away from home (at work or school).

- Type of diet (ovo-lacto vegetarian, 2 g sodium/low-fat diet).
- Foods avoided due to allergy or preference.
- Frequency and dose/amount of medications or nutritional supplements taken daily.
- Satisfaction with diet over a specified time frame (last 3 months, year).

Ⓝ *NCLEX® Connection: Health Promotion and Maintenance, Health Screening*

UNIT 1   PRINCIPLES OF NUTRITION

CHAPTER 4 *Guidelines for Healthy Eating*

Nutrition is vital to maintaining optimal health. Healthy food choices and controlling weight are important steps in promoting health and reducing risk factors for disease.

Nurses should encourage favorable nutritional choices, and can serve as informational resources for clients regarding guidelines for healthy eating.

Established guidelines for healthy eating that clients and nurses can refer to include the Dietary Guidelines for Americans and MyPlate, along with a number of condition- or system-specific guidelines.

Vegetarian diets can meet all nutrients recommendations. It is essential to consume a variety and correct amount of foods to meet individual caloric needs.

DIETARY GUIDELINES FOR AMERICANS

- The U.S. Department of Agriculture (USDA) and the U.S. Department of Health and Human Services (HHS) publish the Dietary Guidelines for Americans jointly every 5 years. These guidelines are based on evidence-based advice concerning food intake and physical activity for Americans older than 2 years of age, including those at risk for chronic disease. The updates can be found on the USDA and health.gov websites.
- The Dietary Guidelines for Americans advocates healthy food selections: a variety of fiber-rich fruits and vegetables, whole grains, low-fat or fat-free milk and milk products, lean meats, poultry, fish, legumes, eggs, and nuts. Recommendations include "nutrient-dense" foods and beverages.
  - Balance energy intake with energy expenditure by selecting a wide variety of foods, and limiting saturated and trans saturated fat, sugars, sodium, and alcohol.
  - Establish exercise routines to promote cardiovascular health, muscle strength and endurance, and psychological well-being.
  - Consume a minimum of five servings per day of fiber-rich fruits and vegetables to in order to decrease risk factors for some cancers. The vitamin and mineral content of these foods can also decrease the risk of DNA damage.
  - Choose monounsaturated and polyunsaturated fats from fish, lean meats, nuts, and vegetable oils. Fat intake can average 30% of total caloric intake with a goal of less than 7% from saturated fats. While progressing toward the 7% goal, individuals should try to consume less than 10% of intake from saturated fats, and progress to 7% or less over time.
  - Limit sugar and starchy foods to decrease the risk of dental caries.
  - Consume less than 2,300 mg/day (about 1 tsp) of salt by limiting most canned and processed foods. Prepare foods without adding salt. Middle-aged and older adults benefit even more from a diet with 1,500 mg/day or less of sodium.
  - Drink alcohol in moderation: up to one drink per day for women and two per day for men. Some medical conditions, medication therapies, and physical activities preclude the use of alcohol.
  - Eating at least 12 oz seafood from a variety of sources is beneficial for individuals older than age 12 years who are not pregnant or nursing. Observe local seafood advisories closely, and limit consumption of large, predatory fish.
  - Follow food safety guidelines when preparing, cooking, and storing food. Avoid consumption of raw eggs and unpasteurized milk and juices. **Q**s

MYPLATE

The USDA sponsors a website that promotes healthy food choices balanced with physical activity (www.choosemyplate.gov). The pyramid is based on the current USDA dietary guidelines, and is a tool to help individuals identify daily amounts of foods based on criteria (age, gender, activity level). The food groups represented are grains, vegetables, fruit, dairy, oils, and protein foods.

MyPlate can serve as a reminder to balance calorie intake with suitable activity.
- Adults should engage in at least 2.5 hr/week of moderate-level aerobic physical activity or 1.25 hr/week of vigorous aerobic physical activity.
- Children and adolescents should be physically active for 60 min/day, the majority of which should be moderate or vigorous aerobic physical activity, but developmentally appropriate and fun. Children should engage in muscle strengthening activities at least 3 days/week. Activity levels can be met in short periods of activity throughout the day instead of a sustained 60 min.

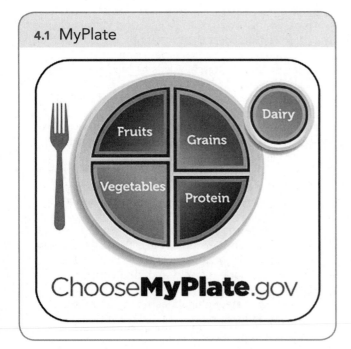

4.1 MyPlate

VEGETARIAN DIETS

- A vegetarian diet focuses on plants for food, including fruits, vegetables, dried beans and peas, grains, seeds, and nuts. There is no single type of vegetarian diet. Vegetarian eating patterns usually fall into the following groups.
  - **Vegan** diet excludes all meat and animal products.
  - **Lacto vegetarian** diet includes dairy products.
  - **Lacto-ovo vegetarian** diet includes dairy products and eggs.
- People who follow vegetarian diets can get all the nutrients they need, but they must be careful to eat a wide variety of foods to meet their nutritional needs. It is important to discuss ensuring enough vitamin D and B$_{12}$, calcium, and omega-3 fatty acids are consumed by clients who follow a vegan diet.

FOOD LABELS

- The Food and Drug Administration (FDA) requires certain information be included with packaged foods and beverages. The information is included on the nutrition facts label or food label, which is a boxed label found on foods and beverages. Food labels must include single serving size, number of servings in the package, percent of daily values, and the amount of each nutrient in one serving.
- The Percent Daily Values information is typically based on a 2,000 calorie/day diet, but for certain nutrients and food components can be based on 2,500 calorie/day.
- Teach clients to read food labels properly to ensure individual nutritional needs are met, and healthy choices are made.
- In July 2015, the FDA recommended changes to the current nutrition facts Label. If approved, labels must be compliant within 2 years of the effective date.

NUTRIENTS INCLUDED ON THE FOOD LABEL
- Calories
- Calories from fat
- Total fat
- Saturated fat
- Trans fat
- Cholesterol
- Sodium
- Total carbohydrates
- Dietary fiber
- Sugars
- Protein
- Vitamin A
- Vitamin C
- Calcium
- Iron

4.2 MyPlate recommended servings

RECOMMENDED DAILY SERVINGS			FOOD SOURCES
Grains			
Whole grains should equal half of the grains eaten.			One slice bread = 1 oz
Children	**Females**	**Males**	1 cup flake cereal = 1 oz
2 to 3 years: 3 oz	9 to 13 years: 5 oz	9 to 13 years: 3 oz	½ cup cooked pasta = 1 oz
4 to 8 years: 5 oz	14 to 50 years: 6 oz	14 to 18 years: 4 oz	1 6-inch flour tortilla = 1 oz
	51 years and older: 5 oz	19 to 30 years: 8 oz	
		31 to 50 years: 7 oz	
		51 years and older: 6 oz	
Vegetables			
Vegetables include raw, cooked, frozen, canned, dried, or 100% juice.			Broccoli, carrots, pumpkin, tomato juice, peas, corn, potatoes, onions, mushrooms
Children	**Females**	**Males**	
2 to 3 years: 1 cup	9 to 13 years: 2 cups	9 to 13 years: 2.5 cups	
4 to 8 years: 1.5 cups	14 to 50 years: 2.5 cups	14 to 50 years: 3 cups	
	51 years and older: 2 cups	51 years and older: 2.5 cups	
Fruits			
Fruits include fresh, frozen, canned, dried, or 100% juice.			One small banana = ½ cup serving
Children	**Females**	**Males**	One small orange = ½ cup serving
2 to 3 years: 1 cup	9 to 18 years: 1.5 cups	9 to 13 years: 1.5 cups	¼ cup dried apricots = ½ cup serving
4 to 8 years: 1 to 1.5 cups	19 to 30 years: 2 cups	14 years and older: 2 cups	
	31 years and older: 1.5 cups		
Dairy			
Dairy selections should include reduced-fat or fat-free options. Higher-fat options are counted as part of daily calories from solid fats and added sugars (i.e., empty calories).			Milk, yogurt, cheese, pudding, ice cream, soy milk
Children	**Females** and **Males**		¼ cup evaporated milk = 1 cup serving
2 to 3 years: 2 cups	9 years and older: 3 cups		½ cup shredded cheese = 1 cup serving
4 to 8 years: 2.5 cups			1.5 oz hard cheese = 1 cup serving
			½ cup ricotta cheese = 1 cup serving
			2 cups cottage cheese = 1 cup serving
			1.5 cups ice cream = 1 cup serving
Proteins			
Protein requirements can increase with physical activity. Selection should include lean or low-fat proteins. Higher fat options are counted as part of daily calories from solid fats and added sugars (i.e., empty calories).			Meats (beef, pork), poultry, eggs, kidney beans, soy beans, seafood, nuts and seeds, peanut butter
Children	**Females**	**Males**	One small chicken breast = 3 oz
2 to 3 years: 2 oz	9 to 18 years: 5 oz	9 to 13 years: 5 oz	1 can drained tuna = 3 to 4 oz
4 to 8 years: 4 oz	19 to 30 years: 5.5 oz	14 to 30 years: 6.5 oz	One egg = 1 oz
	31 years and older: 5 oz	31 to 50 years: 6 oz	¼ cup cooked beans = 1 oz
		51 years and older: 5.5 oz	½ oz seeds or nuts = 1 oz
Oils			
Children	**Females**	**Males**	Vegetable oils (canola, corn, olive, peanut, safflower, soybean, sunflower), mayonnaise, some salad dressings, avocado, nuts and seeds
2 to 3 years: 3 tsp	9 to 18 years: 5 tsp	9 to 13 years: 5 tsp	
4 to 8 years: 4 tsp	19 to 30 years: 6 tsp	14 to 18 year: 6 tsp	Avocados and olives are also part of the vegetable food group.
	31 years and older: 5 tsp	19 to 30 years: 7 tsp	
		31 years and older: 6 tsp	Nuts and seeds are also part of the protein food group.

STRATEGIES FOR PROMOTION OF SPECIFIC AREAS OF HEALTH

Healthy hearts

- Limit saturated fat to 10% of calories and cholesterol to 300 mg/day (with a goal of less than 7% and 200 mg/day).
- For individuals with elevated low density lipoprotein (LDL), the American Heart Association (AHA) recommends increasing monounsaturated fats and soluble fiber.
- The Dietary Approaches to Stop Hypertension (DASH) diet is proven by research to significantly lower systolic and diastolic blood pressure. ○EBP

Healthy nervous systems

- Normal functioning of the nervous system depends on adequate levels of the B-complex vitamins, especially thiamin, niacin, and vitamins B_6 and B_{12}.
- Calcium and sodium are important regulators of nerve responses. Consuming the recommended servings from the grain and dairy food groups provides these nutrients.

Healthy bones

- Consuming the recommended servings from the MyPlate's dairy group supplies the calcium, magnesium, and phosphorus necessary for bone formation.
- Weight-bearing physical activity is essential to decrease the risk of osteoporosis.

Good bowel function

- Normal bowel functioning depends on adequate fluid intake and 25 g/day of fiber for women, and 38 g/day for men.
- The minimum number of servings from MyPlate's fruit, vegetable, and grain food groups (specifically whole grains) provides the essential nutrients.

Cancer prevention

- A well-balanced diet using MyPlate and a healthy weight are guidelines to prevent cancer.
- Increase high-fiber plant-based foods.
- Limit saturated and polyunsaturated fat, while emphasizing foods with monounsaturated fat or omega-3 fatty acids (nuts and fish).
- Limit sodium intake.
- Avoid excess alcohol intake.
- Include regular physical activity.

Application Exercises

1. A nurse is providing teaching to a client who follows vegan dietary practices. The nurse should instruct the client to ensure he is consuming enough of which of the following nutrients? (Select all that apply.)
   - A. Vitamin D
   - B. Fiber
   - C. Calcium
   - D. Vitamin B_{12}
   - E. Whole grains

2. A nurse is conducting a nutrition class to a group of women at a local community center. Which of the following information should the nurse include in the teaching?
   - A. Progress toward limiting saturated fat to 7% of total daily intake.
   - B. Good bowel function requires 35 g/day of fiber for women.
   - C. Limit cholesterol consumption to 400 mg/day.
   - D. Normal functioning cardiac systems depends on B-complex vitamins.

3. A nurse is discussing essential nutrients for normal functioning of the nervous system with a client. Which of the following should the nurse include in the teaching? (Select all that apply.)
   - A. Calcium
   - B. Thiamin
   - C. Vitamin B_6
   - D. Sodium
   - E. Phosphorus

4. A school nurse is teaching a group of students how to read food labels. Which of the following is a required component of food labels that the nurse should include in the teaching? (Select all that apply.)
   - A. Total carbohydrates
   - B. Total fat
   - C. Calories
   - D. Magnesium
   - E. Dietary fiber

PRACTICE Active Learning Scenario

A community health nurse is conducting a nutritional class regarding cancer prevention strategies. Use the ATI Active Learning Template: Basic Concept to complete this item.

RELATED CONTENT: Describe four components recommended to prevent cancer.

Application Exercises Key

1. A. **CORRECT:** The nurse should instruct the client to ensure he is consuming adequate vitamin D because most dietary vitamin D is consumed via fortified milk products. The vegan diet includes plant foods, and excludes all animal-derived products.

   B. Because the vegan diet consists of plant foods, adequate fiber consumption is not a concern. Fiber is found primarily in plants.

   C. **CORRECT:** The nurse should instruct the client to ensure he is consuming adequate vitamin B_{12} because all reliable sources of vitamin B_{12} are in animal products. The vegan diet excludes all animal-derived products.

   D. **CORRECT:** The nurse should instruct the client to monitor and ensure he is consuming adequate calcium because there are few good sources of calcium from plant sources. The vegan diet excludes all animal-derived products.

   E. Because the vegan diet consists of plant foods, adequate consumption of whole grains is not a concern. Grains are included as part of the vegan diet.

   Ⓝ *NCLEX® Connection: Health Promotion and Maintenance, Health Promotion/Disease Prevention*

2. A. **CORRECT:** The nurse should include for the client's to progress toward limiting saturated fat to 7% of total daily intake.

   B. Good bowel function requires 25 g/day of fiber for women, and 38 g/day for men.

   C. Cholesterol consumption should be limited to between 200 and 300 mg/day.

   D. Normal functioning nervous system, instead of cardiac, depends on B-complex vitamins.

   Ⓝ *NCLEX® Connection: Health Promotion and Maintenance, Health Promotion/Disease Prevention*

3. A. **CORRECT:** Calcium is an important regulator of nerve responses.

   B. **CORRECT:** Normal functioning of the nervous system depends on adequate levels of the B-complex vitamins, especially thiamin, niacin, and vitamins B_6 and B_{12}.

   C. **CORRECT:** Normal functioning of the nervous system depends on adequate levels of the B-complex vitamins, especially thiamin, niacin, and vitamins B_6 and B_{12}.

   D. **CORRECT:** Sodium is an important regulator of nerve responses.

   E. Phosphorus helps maintain acid-base balance, as well as formation of bone and teeth, and does not directly affect functioning of the nervous system.

   Ⓝ *NCLEX® Connection: Health Promotion and Maintenance, Health Promotion/Disease Prevention*

4. A. **CORRECT:** The Food and Drug Administration (FDA) requires certain information be included with packaged foods and beverages. Total carbohydrates are included on food labels.

   B. **CORRECT:** Food labels must include single serving size, number of servings in the package, percent of daily values, and the amount of each nutrient in one serving. Total fat is included on food labels.

   C. **CORRECT:** Calories are included on food labels.

   D. Magnesium is not included on food labels.

   E. **CORRECT:** Dietary fiber is included on food labels.

   Ⓝ *NCLEX® Connection: Health Promotion and Maintenance, Aging Process*

PRACTICE Answer

Using the ATI Active Learning Template: Basic Concept

RELATED CONTENT

A well-balanced diet using the MyPlate and a healthy weight are guidelines to prevent cancer.
- Increase high-fiber plant-based foods.
- Limit saturated and polyunsaturated fat, while emphasizing foods with monounsaturated fat or omega-3 fatty acids (nuts and fish).
- Limit sodium intake.
- Avoid excess alcohol intake.
- Include regular physical activity.

Ⓝ *NCLEX® Connection: Health Promotion and Maintenance, Health Promotion/Disease Prevention*

UNIT 1   PRINCIPLES OF NUTRITION

CHAPTER 5   *Food Safety*

Food safety is an important concept in nursing. It is essential to provide clients with the necessary education regarding food safety and food-medication interactions.

Food safety concerns include preventing aspiration of food, reducing the risk of foodborne illness, assessing for food allergies, and understanding food-medication interactions.

FOOD SAFETY GUIDELINES

Ingestion of food poses a risk of aspiration in some circumstances.
- To minimize the risk of aspiration, food should be consumed only by individuals who are conscious and have an intact gag or swallow reflex. Qs
- For clients who have a known risk of aspiration (following a stroke or a procedure involving anesthesia of the esophagus), it is important for nurses to monitor the client's ability to swallow prior to eating.

FOOD SAFETY REQUIREMENTS
- Proper food storage
- Proper handling
- Proper preparation

FOOD STORAGE GUIDELINES

Fresh meat: Maintain refrigerator temperature at 40° F (4° C) or colder.
- **Bacon:** 7 days
- **Sausage** (pork/chicken/beef/turkey): 1 to 2 days
- **Summer sausage:** 3 months (unopened); 3 weeks (opened)
- **Steaks, chops, roasts** (beef, veal, lamb, or pork): 3 to 5 days
- **Chicken or turkey** (whole/parts): 1 to 2 days
- **Fish:** Maintain refrigerator temperature at 40° F (4° C) or colder.
  - Lean or fatty: 1 to 2 days
  - Smoked: 14 days
  - Fresh shellfish: 1 to 2 days
  - Canned: 3 to 4 days (after opening); 5 years (pantry)

Eggs: Store in the refrigerator for 4 to 5 weeks in shell, and 1 week if hard-boiled.

Fruits and vegetables: Refrigerate perishable fruits and vegetables at 40° F (4° C). All pre-cut and pre-peeled fruits and vegetables should also be refrigerated.

Perishables: Do not leave at room temperature for more than 2 hr (1 hr if the temperature is 90° F [32° C] or above).

Canned goods: Check for rusting, crushing, and denting. Observe for stickiness on the outside of can, which may indicate leakage. Do not use any canned foods that are damaged.

HANDLING GUIDELINES
- Wash hands and food preparation surfaces frequently, and before handling food.
- Separate foods to avoid cross-contamination.

PREPARATION GUIDELINES

Cook food to the proper temperature followed by a 3-min rest time.
- Roasts and steaks: 145° F (63° C)
- Chicken: 165° F (74° C)
- Ground beef: 160° F (71° C)
- Products that contain eggs: 160° F (71° C)

PACKAGING LABELS
- **Sell-by date:** The final recommended day of sale.
- **Use-by date:** How long the product will maintain top quality.
- **Expiration date:** The final day the product should be used or consumed.

FOODBORNE ILLNESS

Foodborne illnesses occur due to improper storage of food products, as well as unsafe handling and preparation. In order to decrease the incidence of foodborne illnesses, primary education should be conducted by nurses. Proper handing and preparation is simple and includes performing frequent hand hygiene. It is important to refrigerate food products when necessary, and to avoid cross-contamination when preparing food. Food should be heated to recommended temperatures to kill unwanted bacteria. Following these basic principles can prevent the occurrence of foodborne illnesses. Qs
- Foodborne illnesses pose the greatest risk to children, older adults, immunocompromised clients, and pregnant clients. Ⓖ
- Viruses cause the majority of foodborne illnesses, but bacteria are responsible for the majority of deaths caused by foodborne illness.
- Foods most commonly associated with foodborne illness are the following.
  - Raw or undercooked foods of animal origin
  - Raw fruits and vegetables contaminated with animal feces
  - Raw sprouts
  - Unpasteurized fruit juice
  - Uncooked food handled by someone who is ill

COMMON FOODBORNE ILLNESSES

Salmonella: Occurs due to eating undercooked or raw meat, poultry, eggs, fish, fruit, and dairy products. Common manifestations include headache, fever, abdominal cramping, diarrhea, nausea, and vomiting. This condition can be fatal.

***Escherichia coli* 0157:H7:** Raw or undercooked meat, especially ground beef, can cause this foodborne pathogen. Findings include severe abdominal pain and diarrhea.

Listeria monocytogenes: Soft cheese, raw milk products, undercooked poultry, processed meats, and raw vegetables can cause the illness. *Listeria monocytogenes* causes significant problems for newborns, pregnant clients, and immunocompromised clients. Onset occurs with the development of a sudden fever, diarrhea, headache, back pain, and abdominal discomfort. It can lead to stillbirth or miscarriage.

Norovirus: A viral infection caused by consuming contaminated fruits and vegetables, salads prepared by someone who is infected, oysters, and contaminated water. Norovirus is very contagious, and has an onset of 24 to 48 hr. Manifestations include projectile vomiting, fever, myalgia, watery diarrhea, and headache.

FOOD ALLERGIES

Nutritional assessment/data collection includes identification of food allergies.

- Milk, peanuts, fish, eggs, soy, shellfish, tree nuts and wheat are the most commonly reported food allergies in adults. Some infants my react to cow's milk and/or soy, but typically outgrow this by 4 years of age.
- Common manifestations include nausea, vomiting, diarrhea, abdominal distention, and pain. Some reactions are severe and can cause anaphylaxis.

FOOD-MEDICATION INTERACTIONS

Foods and medications can interact in the body in ways that alter the intended action of medications. The composition and timing of food intake should be considered in relation to medication use.

Foods can alter the absorption of medications.

- **Increased absorption:** Improves the peak effects of some drugs when taken with food.
- **Decreased absorption:** Food can decrease the rate and extent of absorption.
  - Reducing the rate of absorption delays the onset of peak effects.
  - Reducing the extent of absorption reduces the intended effect of the medication.

Some medications cause gastric irritation. It is important to take those medications (ibuprofen, amoxicillin, some antidepressants [bupropion]) with food to avoid gastric upset.

Some foods alter the metabolism/actions of medications. Qs

- Grapefruit juice interferes with the metabolism of many medications, resulting in an increased serum level of the medication.
- Foods high in vitamin K (dark green vegetables, eggs, carrots) can decrease the anticoagulant effects of warfarin.
- Foods high in protein can increase the metabolism of the anti-Parkinson's medication levodopa, which decreases the medication's absorption and amount transported to the brain.
- Tyramine is a naturally occurring amine found in many foods that has hypertensive effects similar to other amines (norepinephrine). Tyramine is metabolized by MAO, and clients taking MAOIs (phenelzine, selegiline) who consume foods high in tyramine can suffer a hypertensive crisis. Foods high in tyramine include aged cheese, smoked meats, dried fish, and overripe avocados.
- Herbal supplements can cause potential interactions with prescribed medications. It is important that any herbal medication consumed by a client be discussed with the provider.

NURSING ASSESSMENT/DATA COLLECTION AND INTERVENTIONS

- Nursing assessments should include a complete dietary profile of the client, medications, herbal supplements, baseline knowledge about food safety, and food-medication interactions.
- Nursing interventions should include basic teaching about food safety, and the interactions between food and client medications.

1. A nurse is providing teaching about food safety and foodborne illness to a group of older adults at a local community center. Which of the following information should the nurse include in the teaching?

    A. "Unpasteurized fruit juice is a common cause of foodborne illness."

    B. "Store hard-boiled eggs in the refrigerator for up to 2 weeks."

    C. "The recommended cooking temperature for ground beef is 145° F."

    D. "The onset of norovirus is 5 to 7 days after exposure to the bacteria."

2. A nurse is providing teaching about food allergies to a group of new parents. The nurse should include that infants who react to which of the following foods typically outgrow the sensitivity? (Select all that apply.)

    A. Soy

    B. Wheat

    C. Cow's milk

    D. Eggs

    E. Fish

3. A nurse is providing teaching to a client who is to begin taking phenelzine. The nurse should include that consuming which of the following foods while taking this medication could cause a hypertensive crisis?

    A. Grapefruit juice

    B. Dark green vegetables

    C. Greek yogurt

    D. Smoked fish

PRACTICE Active Learning Scenario

A nurse is providing teaching to a client about food safety. What should the nurse include in the teaching? Use the ATI Active Learning Template: Basic Concept to complete this item.

UNDERLYING PRINCIPLES
- Describe four food storage guidelines.
- Describe three foodborne illnesses and how they are acquired.

Application Exercises Key

1. A. **CORRECT:** The nurse should include in the teaching that unpasteurized fruit juice is a common cause of foodborne illness. Other common causes of foodborne illness include raw or undercooked foods of animal origin, raw fruits and vegetables contaminated with animal feces, and uncooked food handled by someone who is ill.

    B. The nurse should include in the teaching to store hard-boiled eggs no longer than 1 week.

    C. The nurse should include in the teaching that the recommended cooking temperature for ground beef is 160° F (71° C).

    D. The nurse should include in the teaching that the onset of norovirus is 24 to 48 hr after exposure to the virus.

    (N) *NCLEX® Connection: Health Promotion and Maintenance, Aging Process*

2. A. **CORRECT:** Infants who react to soy typically outgrow the sensitivity by the age of 4 years.

    B. The nurse should include in the teaching that wheat is a common food allergy, but should not include that sensitivities during infancy are typically outgrown later in life.

    C. **CORRECT:** Infants who react to cow's milk typically outgrow the sensitivity by the age of 4 years.

    D. The nurse should include in the teaching that eggs are a common food allergy, but should not include that sensitivities during infancy are typically outgrown later in life.

    E. The nurse should include in the teaching that fish is a common food allergy, but should not include that sensitivities during infancy are typically outgrown later in life.

    (N) *NCLEX® Connection: Health Promotion and Maintenance, Aging Process*

3. A. Grapefruit juice interferes with the metabolism of many medications, but will not cause a hypertensive crisis in the client who is taking phenelzine.

    B. Dark green vegetables can decrease the anticoagulant effects of warfarin, but will not cause a hypertensive crisis in the client who is taking phenelzine.

    C. Greek yogurt is a source of protein that can increase the metabolism of levodopa, but will not cause a hypertensive crisis in the client who is taking phenelzine.

    D. **CORRECT:** Smoked fish is high in tyramine, which has hypertensive effects similar to other amines. Because tyramine is metabolized by MAO, clients who are taking MAOIs, such as phenelzine, and consume tyramine can experience a hypertensive crisis.

    (N) *NCLEX® Connection: Basic Care and Comfort, Nutrition and Oral Hydration*

PRACTICE Answer

Using the ATI Active Learning Template: Basic Concept

UNDERLYING PRINCIPLES

- Proper food storage guidelines
  - Fresh meat: Maintain refrigerator temperature at 40° F (4° C) or colder.
    - Bacon: 7 days
    - Sausage (pork/chicken/beef/turkey): 1 to 2 days
    - Summer sausage: 3 months (unopened); 3 weeks (opened)
    - Steaks, chops, roasts (beef, veal, lamb, or pork): 3 to 5 days
    - Chicken or turkey (whole/parts): 1 to 2 days
  - Fish: Maintain refrigerator temperature at 40° F (4° C) or colder.
    - Lean or fatty: 1 to 2 days
    - Smoked: 14 days
    - Fresh shellfish: 1 to 2 days
    - Canned: 3 to 4 days (after opening); 5 years (pantry)
  - Eggs: Store in the refrigerator for 4 to 5 weeks in shell, and 1 week if hard-boiled.
  - Fruits and vegetables: Refrigerate perishable fruits and vegetables at 40° F (4° C). All pre-cut and pre-peeled fruits and vegetables should also be refrigerated.
  - Do not leave perishables at room temperature for more than 2 hr (1 hr if the temperature is 90° F [32° C] or above)
  - Canned goods: Check for rusting, crushing, and denting. Observe for stickiness on the outside of can, which may indicate leakage. Do not use any canned foods that are damaged.

- Foodborne illnesses
  - Salmonella: Occurs due to eating undercooked or raw meat, poultry, eggs, fish, fruit, and dairy products. Common manifestations include headache, fever, abdominal cramping, diarrhea, nausea, and vomiting. This condition can be fatal.
  - *Escherichia coli* 0157:H7: Raw or undercooked meat, especially ground beef, can cause this foodborne pathogen. Findings include severe abdominal pain and diarrhea.
  - *Listeria monocytogenes:* Soft cheese, raw milk products, undercooked poultry, processed meats, and raw vegetables can cause the illness. *Listeria monocytogenes* causes significant problems for newborns, pregnant clients, and immunocompromised clients. Onset occurs with the development of a sudden fever, diarrhea, headache, back pain, and abdominal discomfort. It can lead to stillbirth or miscarriage.
  - Norovirus: A viral infection caused by consuming contaminated fruits and vegetables, salads prepared by someone who is infected, oysters, and contaminated water. Norovirus is very contagious, and has an onset of 24 to 48 hr. Manifestations include projectile vomiting, fever, myalgia, watery diarrhea, and headache.

(N) *NCLEX® Connection: Health Promotion and Maintenance, Health Promotion/Disease Prevention*

UNIT 1   PRINCIPLES OF NUTRITION

CHAPTER 6 *Cultural, Ethnic, and Religious Influences*

Cultural, ethnic, and religious considerations greatly affect nutritional health. It is imperative that nurses understand cultural needs of clients.

Cultural traditions affect food choices and routines. Nurses should take this into consideration when planning and communicating nutritional goals with clients.

Acculturation is the process of a cultural, ethnic, or religious group's adopting of the dominant culture's behaviors, beliefs, and values.

Nurses must not demonstrate ethnocentrism, which is the belief that one's own cultural practices are the only correct behaviors, beliefs, attitudes, and values.

CULTURE AND NUTRITION

- The degree to which clients follow their cultural, ethnic, or religious group's traditional nutritional practices should guide the nurse's care.
- The first-generation members of a family are more likely to follow their traditional foodway (all aspects of an individual's nutritional practices), with subsequent generations incorporating the host culture's food practices through socialization.
- Frequently, the dominant culture's breakfast and lunch foods are eaten, and traditional meals are consumed at dinner and symbolic events (religious holidays, weddings, childbirth).
- To avoid ethnocentrism, nurses should understand that ideas regarding food choices and nutrition vary among cultures.
  - Beetles and bugs are food items in some cultures.
  - Not all cultures identify with the American ideal of slimness.
  - Milk is not a source of calcium in many cultures (especially when compared to the Mexican-American foodway) due to the high incidence of lactose intolerance.
- Culturally respectful communication is necessary in all forms of client communication, including client education on nutrition.
  - Acceptable eye contact, and touch, and literacy vary among cultures and can affect communication.
  - Americanization of traditional foodways can have positive or negative consequences.
    - New foods are added to the traditional diet.
    - Food dishes are made in new ways.
    - Dietary items might be deleted entirely.

- Religion has a profound influence on foodways, especially because religion crosses geographic boundaries. Implications include the following.
  - Feasting/celebration foods
  - Special food preparations (kosher kitchens in Orthodox Jewish homes)
  - Prescriptive guidelines for animal slaughter (Islam and Orthodox Judaism)
  - Avoidance of stimulants (coffee, tea, caffeinated soda) by Muslims and Mormons
  - Practice of vegetarianism by Seventh-Day Adventists and some Buddhists
  - Fasting for religious holidays (Ramadan for Muslims, or refraining from meat consumption on Ash Wednesday and Fridays during Lent for Catholics)
- Changes in the American foodway reflect cultural changes in American society and present nutritional challenges. Some trends that have made a significant impact on nutrition include the following.
  - Make it quickly.
  - Make it easy and add only three to four ingredients, or pop it ready-made into the microwave.
  - When all else fails, go to the drive-through, order in, or eat out.
- These changes result in diets that are high in salt, carbohydrates, fat, refined sugars, and caffeine while providing low amounts of fiber and calcium.
- Paying careful attention to reading labels, adding beneficial side dishes, practicing portion control, and choosing better dine-out options can minimize the detrimental effect of societal changes.

VEGETARIAN DIETS

Vegan
- Individuals following a pure vegan diet do not consume animal products of any type, including eggs and milk products. These diets are often adequate in protein due to the intake of nuts and legumes (dried peas and cooked beans). Vitamin B_{12} and vitamin D supplementation might be needed with a pure vegan diet.
- A pure vegan diet requires that a variety of plant materials be consumed in specific combinations in order to ensure essential amino acid intake.

Lacto vegetarian: Individuals following this diet consume milk products in addition to plant-based products.

Ovo-lacto vegetarian: Individuals following this diet consume milk products and eggs in addition to plant-based products.

Ovo vegetarian: Individuals following this diet consume eggs in addition to plant-based products.

SELECTED CULTURAL SUBGROUPS

African American ("soul food")

Origins in the Caribbean, Central America, East Africa, and West Africa

TRADITIONAL FOODS: Rice, grits, cornbread, hominy, okra, greens, sweet potatoes, apples, peaches, buttermilk, pudding, cheddar or American cheese, ham, pork, chicken, catfish, black-eyed peas, red and pinto beans, peanuts, soft drinks, fatback, chitterlings, banana pudding

TRADITIONAL FOOD PREPARATION
- Frying and cooking with added animal fats (lard, salt pork)
- Promoting a shared inheritance and loving family

ACCULTURATION
- Increased milk consumption
- Use of packaged meat, pork preferred
- Continued low intake of fruit and vegetables

NUTRITIONAL HEALTH RISKS
- High in fat, protein, and sodium
- Low in potassium, calcium, and fiber
- Low fresh fruit and vegetable intake
- Substantial weight equated with good health and prosperity
- Increased incidence of type 2 diabetes mellitus, heart disease, and hypertension

HEALTH PROMOTION
- Encourage frying lightly with canola/olive oil instead of animal fats.
- Introduce fresh fruit and vegetable dishes, and decrease meat portions.
- Suggest dark green leafy vegetables and low-fat cheeses as calcium sources.
- Associate "good health" with better food choices and portion control.
- Advise preparing unhealthy soul food items only at special occasions.

Asian American ("Chinese food")

Origins in the Far East, Southeast Asia, and the Indian subcontinent

TRADITIONAL FOODS: Wheat (northern), rice (southern), noodles, fruits, land and sea vegetables, nuts/seeds, soy foods (tofu), nut/seed oils, fish, shellfish, poultry, eggs, sweets, rarely red meats, tea, beer

TRADITIONAL FOOD PREPARATION
- Fruits and vegetables peeled and raw
- Stir-frying in oils quickly to retain crispness of vegetables
- Cutting meat and poultry into bite-sized pieces
- Cooking with salt, oil, and oil products (spices important)
- Preventing imbalances and indigestion through balance of yin and yang

ACCULTURATION
- Increased use of bread and cereal; rice/wheat staple remains high
- Use of new location's fruit and vegetables with increased use of fruit and salads
- Increased use of sugar through soft drinks, candy, and desserts

NUTRITIONAL HEALTH RISKS
- High sodium intake
- Increased cancer rate as living in the U.S. continues

HEALTH PROMOTION
- Encourage continued use of plant-based diet and food preparation as generations take on "American foods."
- Moderate salt intake.
- Limit sugar-laden foods.

Latino American ("Mexican food")

Origins in Mexico, Caribbean, and Central and South America

TRADITIONAL FOODS: Rice, maize, tortillas, tropical fruits, vegetables, nuts, beans, legumes, eggs, cheese, seafood, poultry, infrequent sweets and red meat

TRADITIONAL FOOD PREPARATION
- Frying and stewing in lard or oil
- Meats ground or chopped
- Meat mixed with vegetables and grains, or stuffed (tamales)
- Heavily spiced with common use of chilies
- Minimal use of sugar
- "Hot" and "cold" food choices maintain balance

ACCULTURATION
- Increased milk use
- Decreased meat consumption as mixed meals decline
- Replacement of maize by wheat in tortillas and breads
- Decreased bean use and change in rice preparation to plain boiled rice
- Increased fruit and vegetable intake
- Added fats in the form of butter or salad dressings on cooked vegetables and side salads
- Replacement of fruit-based drinks by sugar-laden drinks

NUTRITIONAL HEALTH RISKS
- Increased incidence of type 2 diabetes mellitus
- Positive associations with substantial weight

HEALTH PROMOTION
- Encourage boiling, braising, and baking in place of frying and stewing in lard and oils.
- Return to traditional corn tortillas.
- Encourage use of fresh unprocessed/preserved plant-based diet.

Application Exercises

1. A nurse is assisting a client with selecting food choices on a menu. Which of the following actions by the nurse demonstrates ethnocentricity?

    A. Asking the client what he likes to eat

    B. Notifying the dietitian to complete the menu

    C. Recommending one's own favorite foods

    D. Asking the client's family to fill out the menu

2. A nurse is caring for an Asian client who has hypertension. Which of the traditional Asian dietary patterns places the client at risk for this condition?

    A. Incorporation of plant based foods in the diet

    B. Consumption of raw fruits

    C. Preparation of foods using sodium

    D. Focus on shellfish in the diet

3. A nurse educator is teaching a class on culture and food to a group of newly hired nurses. Which of the following statements by a nurse indicates an understanding of the teaching?

    A. "Clients who practice Roman Catholicism do not drink caffeinated beverages."

    B. "Clients who practice orthodox Judaism do not eat meat with daily products."

    C. "Clients who are Mormon eat only the protein of animals that are slaughtered under strict guidelines."

    D. "Clients who practice Hinduism do not eat dairy products."

4. A nurse is caring for a client who follows a vegan diet. Which of the following foods should the nurse offer the client?

    A. Bagel with cream cheese

    B. Fried egg

    C. Fruit with yogurt

    D. Wheat toast with peanut butter

PRACTICE Active Learning Scenario

A nurse is providing teaching to a Latin American client on nutrition. What cultural considerations should guide the nurse with the teaching? Use the ATI Active Learning Template: Basic Concept to complete this item to include the following.

RELATED CONTENT

- Traditional food preparation: Describe four characteristics in the Latin culture.
- Acculturation: Describe three examples among Latinos living in the U.S.
- Health risks: Describe two risks related to the Latin American diet.

Application Exercises Key

1. A. Asking the client what he likes to eat demonstrates sensitivity to the client's food preferences.

   B. Calling the dietitian to fill out the menu does not demonstrate sensitivity to the client's food preferences. However, it is not an example of an ethnocentric approach.

   C. **CORRECT:** Recommending one's own favorite foods is an example of ethnocentrism, which is the belief that one's own cultural practices are the only correct behaviors/beliefs.

   D. Having the family fill out the menu does not demonstrate sensitivity to the client's food preferences. However, it is not an example of an ethnocentric approach.

   Ⓝ *NCLEX® Connection: Psychosocial Integrity, Cultural Awareness/Cultural Influences on Health*

2. A. The nurse should encourage plant-based foods to increase nutrients in the diet.

   B. The nurse should encourage raw fruits in the client's diet to increased vitamin intake.

   C. **CORRECT:** The preparation of foods using sodium places the client at risk for hypertension. Many spices in the Asian diet contain sodium, or it is used as a preservative. The client should reduce sodium consumption.

   D. The nurse should encourage the consumption of shellfish because it is a good source of protein and vitamins.

   Ⓝ *NCLEX® Connection: Health Promotion and Maintenance, High Risk Behaviors*

3. A. This is not a practice of Roman Catholics. Caffeinated beverages are not consumed by Mormons and Muslims because caffeine is a stimulant.

   B. **CORRECT:** Clients who practice Orthodox Judaism do not eat meat with daily products.

   C. Clients who follow the teachings of Islam eat only the protein of animals that are slaughtered under strict guidelines.

   D. Clients who practice Hinduism believe dairy products enhance spiritual purity.

   Ⓝ *NCLEX® Connection: Health Promotion and Maintenance, High Risk Behaviors*

4. A. A client who follows a vegan diet does not eat animal products, such as cream cheese.

   B. A client who follows a vegan diet does not eat animal products, such as a fried egg.

   C. A client who follows a vegan diet does not eat animal products, such as yogurt.

   D. **CORRECT:** A client who follows a vegan diet does not eat animal products. Peanut butter and wheat bread are plant-based.

   Ⓝ *NCLEX® Connection: Psychosocial Integrity, Cultural Awareness/Cultural Influences on Health*

PRACTICE Answer

Using the ATI Active Learning Template: Basic Concept

RELATED CONTENT

- Traditional food preparation
  - Frying and stewing in lard or oil
  - Meats are ground or chopped
  - Meat is mixed with vegetables and grains, or stuffed (tamales)
  - Heavily spiced with common use of chilies
  - Minimal use of sugar
  - "Hot" and "cold" food choices maintain balance
- Acculturation
  - Increased milk use
  - Decreased meat consumption as mixed meals decline
  - Replacement of maize by wheat in tortillas and breads
  - Decreased bean use and change in rice preparation to plain boiled rice
  - Increased fruit and vegetable intake
  - Added fats in the form of butter or salad dressings on cooked vegetables and side salads
  - Replacement of fruit-based drinks by sugar-laden drinks
- Health risks
  - Increased incidence of type 2 diabetes mellitus
  - Positive associations with substantial weight

Ⓝ *NCLEX® Connection: Psychosocial Integrity, Cultural Awareness/Cultural Influences on Health*

UNIT 1   PRINCIPLES OF NUTRITION

CHAPTER 7 *Nutrition Across the Lifespan*

Nutritional needs change as clients pass through the stages of the lifespan, reflecting physiological changes.

Nurses must address nutritional needs across the lifespan and have a thorough understanding of how needs change. Nurses should focus on planning and implementing dietary plans that meet clients' specific needs.

Major stages of the lifespan that have specific nutritional needs include pregnancy and lactation; infancy; childhood; adolescence; and adulthood and older adulthood. ©

Pregnancy and lactation

- Prepregnancy nutrition is highly significant and plays an important role, because early fetal development occurs before a woman might realize she is pregnant. A woman should be well nourished and within her normal weight range prior to conception.
- Good nutrition during pregnancy is essential for the health of the unborn child.
- Maternal nutritional demands are increased for the development of the placenta, enlargement of the uterus, formation of amniotic fluid, increase in blood volume, and preparation of the breasts for lactation.
- A daily increase of 340 calories is recommended during the second trimester of pregnancy, and an increase of 452 calories is recommended during the third trimester of pregnancy.
- The nutritional requirements of women who are pregnant or lactating involves more than increased caloric intake. Specific dietary requirements for major nutrients and micronutrients should be met.

DIETARY GUIDELINES

- Achieving an appropriate amount of weight gain during pregnancy prepares a woman for the energy demands of labor and lactation, and contributes to the delivery of a newborn of normal birth weight.
- The recommended weight gain during pregnancy varies for each woman depending on her body mass index (BMI) and weight prior to pregnancy. **(7.1)**
- Lactating women require an increase in daily caloric intake. If the client is breastfeeding during the postpartum period, an additional daily intake of 330 calories is recommended during the first 6 months, and an additional daily intake of 400 calories is recommended during the second 6 months.

MAJOR AND MICRONUTRIENT REQUIREMENTS

- Dietary requirements for major nutrients
  - Protein should comprise 20% of the daily total calorie intake. The Dietary Reference Intake (DRI) for protein during pregnancy is 1.1 g/kg/day. Protein is essential for rapid tissue growth of maternal and fetal structures, amniotic fluid, and extra blood volume. Women who are pregnant should be aware that animal sources of protein might contain large amounts of fats.
  - Fat should be limited to 30% of total daily calorie intake.
  - Carbohydrates should comprise 50% of the total daily calorie intake. Ensuring adequate carbohydrate intake allows for protein to be spared and available for the synthesis of fetal tissue.
- The need for most vitamins and minerals increases during pregnancy and lactation. Vitamins are essential for blood formation, absorption of iron, and development of fetal tissue. **TABLE 7.2** lists the comparative dietary reference intakes (DRIs) of major vitamins for women age 19 to 30 during nonpregnancy, pregnancy, and lactation.

7.1 Recommended weight gain during pregnancy

FIRST TRIMESTER: Recommended weight gain is 1.1 to 4.4 lb.

SECOND AND THIRD TRIMESTERS: Recommended weight gain is 2 to 4 lb/month.
- **Normal weight client (BMI 18.5–24.9):** 1 lb/week for a total of 25 to 35 lb.
- **Underweight client (BMI < 18.5):** just more than 1 lb/week for a total of 28 to 40 lb.
- **Overweight client (BMI 25–29.9):** 0.66 lb/week for a total of 15 to 25 lb.
- **Obese client (BMI > 30):** 0.5 lb/week for a total of 11 to 20 lb.

ADDITIONAL DIETARY RECOMMENDATIONS

Fluid: 2,000 to 3,000 mL fluids daily from food and drinks. Preferred fluids include water, fruit juice, and milk. Carbonated beverages and fruit drinks provide little or no nutrients.

Alcohol: It is recommended that women abstain from alcohol consumption during pregnancy.

Caffeine: Caffeine crosses the placenta and can affect the movement and heart rate of the fetus. However, moderate use (less than 300 mg/day) does not appear to be harmful.

Vegetarian diets: Well-balanced vegetarian diets that include dairy products can provide all the nutritional requirements of pregnancy.

Folic acid intake: It is recommended that 600 mcg/day of folic acid be taken during pregnancy. Current recommendations for lactating clients include 500 mcg/day folic acid. It is necessary for the neurological development of the fetus and to prevent birth defects. It is essential for maternal red blood cell formation. Food sources include green leafy vegetables, enriched grains, and orange juice.

Iron: The DRI for iron increases by 50% during pregnancy to support the increase in maternal blood volume and to provide iron for fetal liver storage. Iron can be obtained from dairy products and meats, especially red meats. Consuming foods high in vitamin C aids in the absorption of iron. It is recommended that pregnant women take a supplement of 27 mg iron daily to assure adequate intake.

Fish: The FDA has issued advisories regarding fish and shellfish consumption during pregnancy due to the risk of mercury levels. Mercury can be toxic to developing fetal brain tissue.

DIETARY COMPLICATIONS

Nausea and constipation are common during pregnancy.
- For nausea, eat dry crackers or toast. Avoid alcohol, caffeine, fats, and spices. Avoid drinking fluids with meals, and do not take medications to control nausea without checking with the provider.
- For constipation, increase fluid consumption (at least 8 cups per day) and include extra fiber in the diet. Fruits, vegetables, and whole grains contain fiber.

Maternal phenylketonuria (PKU) is a maternal genetic disease in which high levels of phenylalanine pose danger to the fetus.
- It is important for a client to start the PKU diet at least 3 months prior to pregnancy, and continue the diet throughout pregnancy.
- The diet should include foods low in phenylalanine. Foods high in protein (fish, poultry, meat, eggs, nuts, dairy products) must be avoided due to high phenylalanine levels. Q_s
- The client's blood phenylalanine levels should be monitored during pregnancy.
- These interventions will prevent fetal complications (intellectual disability, behavioral problems).

ASSESSMENT/DATA COLLECTION AND INTERVENTIONS

- Nursing assessments should include a complete profile of the client's knowledge base regarding nutritional requirements during pregnancy.
- Nurses should review the recommended dietary practices for pregnant and lactating women with the client, while providing materials containing this information.

Infancy

- Growth rate during infancy is more rapid than any other period of the life cycle. It is important to understand normal growth patterns to determine the adequacy of an infant's nutritional intake.
- Birth weight doubles by 4 to 6 months and triples by 1 year of age. The need for calories and nutrients is high to support the rapid rate of growth.
- Appropriate weight gain averages 0.15 to 0.21 kg (5 to 7 oz) per week during the first 5 to 6 months.
- An infant grows approximately 2.5 cm (1 in) per month in height during the first 6 months, and approximately 1.25 cm (0.5 in) per month during the second 6 months.
- Head circumference increases rapidly during the first 6 months at a rate of 1.5 cm (0.6 in) per month. The rate slows to 0.5 cm/month for months 6 to 12. By 1 year, head size should have increased by 33%. This is reflective of the growth of the nervous system.

7.2 DRIs of major vitamins

NUTRIENT	NONPREGNANT	PREGNANT	LACTATING
Protein	46 g	71 g	71 g
Vitamin A	700 mcg	770 mcg	1,300 mcg
Vitamin C	75 mg	85 mg	120 mg
Vitamin D*	15 mcg	15 mcg	15 mcg
Vitamin E	15 mcg	15 mcg	19 mcg
Vitamin K*	90 mcg	90 mcg	90 mcg
Thiamin	1.1 mg	1.4 mg	1.4 mg
Vitamin B$_6$	1.3 mg	1.9 mg	2.0 mg
Folate	400 mcg	600 mcg	500 mcg
Vitamin B$_{12}$	2.4 mcg	2.6 mcg	2.8 mcg
Calcium*	1,000 mg	1,000 mg	1,000 mg
Iron	18 mg	27 mg	9 mg

*Values represent adequate intakes.

Source: Office of Dietary Supplements. National Institutes of Health, ods.od.nih.gov

- Breast milk, infant formula, or a combination of the two is the sole source of nutrition for the first 4 to 6 months of life. Currently, the American Academy of Pediatrics (AAP) recommends exclusive breastfeeding for the first 6 months of life, followed by breastfeeding with the introduction of complementary foods until at least 12 months of age, then continuation of breastfeeding for as long as the mother and infant desire.
- Semisolid foods should not be introduced before 4 months of age to coincide with the development of head control, ability to sit, and the back-and-forth motion of the tongue.
- Iron-fortified infant cereal is the first solid food introduced as gestational iron stores begin to deplete around 4 months of age.
- Cow's milk should not be introduced into the diet until after 1 year of age because protein and mineral content stress the immature kidney. A young infant cannot fully digest the protein and fat contained in cow's milk.

MEETING NUTRITIONAL NEEDS

BREASTFEEDING

- The AAP recommends that infants receive breast milk for the first 6 to 12 months of age (exclusive breast feeding). Even a short period of breastfeeding has physiological benefits.
- Donor milk may be considered in certain circumstances.
  - The choice to feed an infant human milk from a source other than the infant's mother should be made in consultation with the provider, because the nutritional needs of each infant depend on many factors, including the infant's age and health.
  - The FDA recommends that if an infant is to be fed human milk from a source other than the infant's mother, use only milk from a source that has screened its donors and take other precautions to ensure the safety of the milk. Qs
- Joint Commission National Quality Measures include the following perinatal care measures.
  - Exclusive breast milk feeding during the newborn's entire hospitalization
  - Exclusive breast milk feeding during the newborn's entire hospitalization, considering mother's choice
  - The rationale for these measures are that exclusive breast milk feeding for the first 6 months of neonatal life has long been the expressed goal of World Health Organization (WHO), Department of Health and Human Services (HHS), AAP, and American College of Obstetricians and Gynecologists.
- The AAP recommends that for the first 6 months, infants should receive no water or formula except in cases of medical indication or informed parental choice. In the hospital, no water or formula should be given to a breastfed infant unless prescribed by a provider. QEBP

Advantages of breastfeeding

- Incidence of otitis media (ear infections), type 1 and type 2 diabetes mellitus, obesity, leukemia, lymphoma, and gastrointestinal and respiratory disorders are reduced. This is due to the transfer of antibodies from mother to infant.
- Carbohydrates, proteins, and fats in breast milk are predigested for ready absorption.
- Breast milk is high in omega-3 fatty acids.
- Breast milk is low in sodium.
- Iron, zinc, and magnesium found in breast milk are highly absorbable.
- Calcium absorption is enhanced, as the calcium-to-phosphorous ratio is 2:1.
- The risk of allergies is reduced.
- Maternal-infant bonding is promoted.

Breastfeeding teaching points

- The newborn is offered the breast immediately after birth and frequently thereafter. There should be eight to 12 feedings in a 24-hr period.
- Instruct the mother to demand-feed the infant and to assess for hunger cues. These include rooting, suckling on hands and fingers, and rapid eye movement. Crying is a late indicator of hunger.
- The newborn should nurse up to 15 to 20 min per breast. However, avoid educating clients regarding an expected duration of feedings. Clients should be educated on how to evaluate when the newborn has completed the feeding by noting the slowing of newborn suckling, a softened breast, or sleeping. QEBP
- Do not offer the newborn any supplements unless indicated by the provider.
- The mother's milk supply is equal to the demand of the infant.
- Eventually, the infant will empty a breast within 5 to 10 min, but might need to continue to suck to meet comfort needs.
- Frequent feedings (every 2 hr may be indicated) and manual expression of milk to initiate flow can be needed.
- If it has been 4 hr and the infant has not breastfed, the mother should awaken the infant for feeding.
- Every effort will be made to encourage mothers to express breast milk for supplementation if extra fluids or calories are required.
- Expressed milk can be refrigerated in sterile bottles or storage bags and labeled with the date and time the milk was expressed. It can be maintained in the refrigerator for 10 days or frozen in sterile containers for 6 months.
- Thaw milk in the refrigerator. It can be stored for 24 hr after thawing. Defrosting or heating in a microwave oven is not recommended because high heat destroys some of milk's antibodies, and can burn the infant's oral mucosa.
- Do not refreeze thawed milk.

- Unused breast milk must be discarded.
- Avoid consuming freshwater fish or alcohol, and limit caffeine.
- Instruct the mother to begin manual expression of her breast or use an electric breast pump if the infant is unable to breastfeed due to prematurity or respiratory distress.
- Do not take medications unless prescribed by a provider.

FORMULA FEEDING

Can be used in place of breastfeeding, as an occasional supplement to breastfeeding, or when exclusively breastfed infants are weaned before 12 months of age.

- No artificial pacifier or bottles should be used until after 2 weeks and when breastfeeding is well established.
- Commercial infant formulas provide an alternative to breast milk. They are modified from cow's milk to provide comparable nutrients. However, breast milk is far superior to any formula and even more crucial for a premature infant.
- An iron-fortified formula is recommended by the AAP for at least the first 6 months of life or until the infant consumes adequate solid food. After 6 months, formula without added iron might be indicated.
- Fluoride supplements can be required if an adequate level is not supplied by the water supply.
- Wash hands prior to preparing formula.
- Precisely follow the manufacturer's mixing directions.
- Bottles of mixed formula or open cans of liquid formula require refrigeration. Do not use if the formula has been left at room temperature for 2 hr or longer. Do not reuse partially emptied bottles of formula.
- Formula may be fed chilled, warmed, or at room temperature. Always give formula at approximately the same temperature.
- Hold the infant during feedings with the head slightly elevated to facilitate passage of formula into the stomach. Tilt the bottle to maintain formula in the nipple and prevent the swallowing of air.
- Do not prop the bottle or put an infant to bed with a bottle. This practice promotes tooth decay.
- The infant should not drink more than 32 oz formula per 24 hr period unless directed by a provider.

WEANING

- Developmentally, the infant is ready for weaning from the breast or bottle to a cup between 5 to 8 months of age.
- If breastfeeding is eliminated before 5 to 6 months, a bottle should be provided for the infant's sucking needs.
- It is best to substitute the cup for one feeding period at a time over 5 to 7 days.
- Nighttime feedings are often the last to disappear.
- Never allow a child to take a bottle to bed, as this promotes dental caries.
- Use the new schedule for a second feeding period and continue at the infant's pace.
- The infant might not be ready to wean from the bottle or breast until 12 to 14 months of age.

INTRODUCING SOLID FOOD

- Solid food should not be introduced before 4 to 6 months of age due to the risk of food allergies and stress on the immature kidneys. The AAP prefers introduction of solids foods after 6 months of age. Qs
- Indicators for readiness include voluntary control of the head and trunk, hunger less than 4 hr after vigorous nursing or intake of 8 oz of formula, and interest of the infant.
- Iron-fortified rice cereal should be offered first. Wheat cereals should not be introduced until after the first year. Do not put cereal in the infant's bottle.
- New foods should be introduced one at a time over a 5- to 7-day period to observe for indications of allergy or intolerance, which can include fussiness, rash, upper respiratory distress, vomiting, diarrhea, or constipation. The order of introduction of new foods is no longer considered important, and meat may be introduced first due to its iron and zinc content. QEBP
- Delay the introduction of milk, eggs, wheat, and citrus fruits that can lead to allergic reactions in susceptible infants.
- Do not give peanuts or peanut butter due to the risk of a severe allergic reaction.
- The infant can be ready for three meals per day with three snacks by 8 months of age.
- Homemade baby food is an acceptable feeding option. Do not use canned or packaged foods that are high in sodium. Select fresh or frozen foods, and do not add sugars or other seasonings.
- Open jars of infant food can be stored in the refrigerator for up to 24 hr.
- By 9 months of age, the infant should be able to eat table foods that are cooked, chopped, and unseasoned.
- Do not feed the infant honey due to the risk of botulism.
- Appropriate finger foods include ripe bananas, toast strips, graham crackers, cheese cubes, noodles, and peeled chunks of apples, pears, or peaches.

SUGGESTED INTRODUCTION OF FOODS
- Birth to 4 months: Breast milk (until 6 months) or formula (at 4 months)
- 4 to 6 months: Iron-fortified rice cereal
- 6 to 8 months: Vegetables, fruits or strained meats
- 8 to 10 months: Fish, poultry
- 9 to 12 months: Table foods (cooked, chopped, and unseasoned)
- 12 months: Cow's milk, eggs, cheese

NUTRITION-RELATED PROBLEMS

Colic

Colic is characterized by persistent crying lasting 3 hr or longer per day.
- The cause of colic is unknown, but usually occurs in the late afternoon, more than 3 days per week for more than 3 weeks. The crying is accompanied by a tense abdomen and legs drawn up to the belly.
- Colic usually resolves by 3 months of age.
- Breastfeeding mothers should continue nursing, but limit caffeine and nicotine intake.
- If breastfeeding, eliminating cruciferous vegetables (cauliflower, broccoli, and Brussels sprouts), cow's milk, onion, and chocolate can be helpful.
- Burp the infant in an upright position.
- Other comforting techniques (swaddling, carrying the infant, rocking, repetitive soft sound) can soothe the infant.
- Most infants grow and gain weight despite colic.
- Reassure the parent that colic is transient and does not indicate more serious problems or a lack of parental ability. Qpcc

Lactose intolerance

Lactose intolerance is the inability to digest significant amounts of lactose (the predominant sugar of milk) and is due to inadequate lactase (the enzyme that digests lactose into glucose and galactose).
- Lactose intolerance has an increased prevalence in individuals of Asian, Native American, African, Latino, and Mediterranean descent.
- Clinical findings include abdominal distention, flatus, and occasional diarrhea.
- Soy-based or casein hydrolysate formulas can be prescribed as alternative formulas for infants who are lactose intolerant.

Failure to thrive

Failure to thrive is defined as inadequate gains in weight and height in comparison to established growth and development norms.
- Assess for clinical findings of congenital defects, central nervous system disorders, or partial intestinal obstruction.
- Monitor for swallowing or sucking problems.
- Identify feeding patterns, especially concerning preparation of formulas.
- Observe for psychosocial problems, especially parent-infant bonding, abuse/neglect.
- Provide supportive nutritional guidance. Usually a high-calorie, high-protein diet is indicated.
- Provide supportive parenting guidance.

Diarrhea

Diarrhea is characterized by the passage of more than three loose, watery stools over a 24-hr period.
- Overfeeding and food intolerances are common causes of osmotic diarrhea.
- Infectious diarrhea in the infant is commonly caused by rotavirus.
- Mild diarrhea can require no specific interventions. Check with the provider for any diet modifications.
- Treatment for moderate diarrhea should begin at home with oral rehydration solutions. After each loose stool, 8 oz solution should be given. Sports drinks are contraindicated.
- Educate parents about the clinical findings of dehydration: listlessness, sunken eyes, sunken fontanels, decreased tears, dry mucous membranes, and decreased urine output.
- Breastfed infants should continue nursing.
- Formula-fed infants usually do not require diluted formulas or special formulas.
- Contact the provider if clinical findings of dehydration are present, or if vomiting, bloody stools, high fever, change in mental status, or refusal to take liquids occurs.

Constipation

Constipation is the inability or difficulty to evacuate the bowels.
- Constipation is not a common problem for breastfed infants.
- Constipation can be caused by formula that is too concentrated or by inadequate carbohydrate intake.
- Stress the importance of accurate dilution of formula.
- Advise adherence to the recommended amount of formula intake for age.

NURSING ASSESSMENT/DATA COLLECTION AND INTERVENTIONS

- Nursing assessments should include an assessment of knowledge base of the client regarding nutritional guidelines for infants, normal infant growth patterns, breastfeeding, formula feeding, and the progression for the introduction of solid foods.
- Additionally, nurses should provide education and references for the client regarding each of the assessments listed above.

Childhood

- Growth rate slows following infancy.
- ChooseMyPlate.gov is a food guidance system that offers an Internet-based tool to provide clients with individualized recommendations for adequate nutrition. Children require the same food groups as adults, but in smaller serving sizes. SuperTracker can be used to create an individualized plan based on age, gender, and body composition. Q↳
- Energy needs and appetite vary with the child's activity level.
- Generally, nutrient needs increase with age.
- Attitudes toward food and general food habits are established by 5 years of age.
- Increasing the variety and texture of foods helps the child develop good eating habits.
- Foods like hot dogs, popcorn, peanuts, grapes, raw carrots, celery, peanut butter, tough meat, and candy can cause choking or aspiration. Qs
- Inclusion in family mealtime is important for social development.
- Group eating becomes a significant means of socialization for school-age children.

TODDLERS: 1 TO 3 YEARS OLD

NUTRITION GUIDELINES

- Toddlers generally grow 2 to 3 inches in height and gain approximately 5 lb/year.
- Limit 100% juice to 4 to 6 oz a day.
- The 1- to 2-year-old child requires whole cow's milk to provide adequate fat for the still-growing brain.
- Food serving size is 1 tbsp for each year of age.
- Exposure to a new food might be needed 8 to 15 times before the child develops an acceptance of it.
- If there is a negative family history for allergies, cow's milk, chocolate, citrus fruits, egg white, seafood, and nut butters may be gradually introduced while monitoring the child for reactions.
- Toddlers prefer finger foods because of their increasing autonomy. They prefer plain foods to mixtures, but usually like macaroni and cheese, spaghetti, and pizza.
- Regular meal times and nutritious snacks best meet nutrient needs.
- Snacks or desserts that are high in sugar, fat, or sodium should be avoided.
- Children are at an increased risk for choking until 4 years of age.
- Avoid foods that are potential choking hazards. Always provide adult supervision during snack and mealtimes. During food preparation, cut small, bite-sized pieces that are easy to swallow to prevent choking. Do not allow the child to engage in drinking or eating during play activities or while lying down. Qs

NUTRITIONAL CONCERNS/RISKS

Iron

- Iron deficiency anemia is the most common nutritional deficiency disorder in children.
- Lean red meats provide sources of readily absorbable iron.
- Consuming vitamin C (orange juice, tomatoes) with plant sources of iron (beans, raisins, peanut butter, whole grains) will maximize absorption.
- Milk should be limited to the recommended quantities (24 oz) because it is a poor source of iron and can displace the intake of iron-rich foods.

Vitamin D

- Vitamin D is essential for bone development.
- Recommended vitamin D intake is the same (5 mcg/day) from birth through age 50. Children require more vitamin D because their bones are growing.
- Milk (cow, soy) and fatty fish are good sources of vitamin D.
- Sunlight exposure leads to vitamin D synthesis. Children who spend large amounts of time inside (watching TV, playing video games) are at an increased risk for vitamin D deficiency.
- Vitamin D assists in the absorption of calcium into the bones.

PRESCHOOLERS: 3 TO 6 YEARS

NUTRITION GUIDELINES

- Preschoolers generally grow 2 to 3 inches in height and gain approximately 5 lb/year.
- Preschoolers need 13 to 19 g/day of complete protein in addition to adequate calcium, iron, folate, and vitamins A and C.
- Preschoolers tend to dislike strong-tasting vegetables (cabbage, onions), but like many raw vegetables that are eaten as finger foods.
- Food jags (ritualistic preference for one food) are common and usually short-lived.
- MyPlate guidelines are appropriate, requiring the lowest number of servings per food group.
- Food patterns and preferences are first learned from the family, and peers begin influencing preferences and habits at around 5 years of age.

NUTRITIONAL CONCERNS/RISKS

Concerns include overfeeding; intake of high-calorie, high-fat, high-sodium snacks, soft drinks, and juices; and inadequate intake of fruits and vegetables.

- Be alert to the appropriate serving size of foods (1 tbsp per year of age).
- Avoid high-fat and high-sugar snacks.
- Encourage daily physical activities.
- May switch to skim or 1% low-fat milk after 2 years of age.

Iron deficiency anemia

Lead poisoning is a risk for children younger than 6 years of age because they frequently place objects in their mouths that can contain lead, and have a higher rate of intestinal absorption.

- Feed children at frequent intervals because more lead is absorbed on an empty stomach. **Qs**
- Inadequate intake of calories, calcium, iron, zinc, and phosphorous can increase susceptibility.

SCHOOL-AGE CHILDREN: 6 TO 12 YEARS

NUTRITION GUIDELINES

- School-age children generally grow 2 to 3 inches in height and gain approximately 5 lb/year.
- Following MyPlate recommendations, the diet should provide variety, balance, and moderation.
- Young athletes need to meet energy, protein, and fluid needs.
- Educate children to make healthy food selections.
- Children enjoy learning how to safely prepare nutritious snacks.
- Children need to learn to eat snacks only when hungry, not when bored or inactive.

NUTRITIONAL CONCERNS/RISKS

Skipping breakfast occurs in about 10% of children.

- Optimum performance in school is dependent on a nutritious breakfast.
- Children who regularly eat breakfast tend to have an age-appropriate BMI.

Overweight/obesity affects at least 20% of children.

- Greater psychosocial implications exist for children than adults.
- Overweight children tend to be obese adults.
- Prevention is essential. Encourage healthy eating habits, decrease fats and sugars (empty-calorie foods), and increase the level of physical activity.
- A weight-loss program directed by a provider is indicated for children who are more than 40% overweight.
- Praise the child's abilities and skills.
- Never use food as a reward or punishment.

NURSING ASSESSMENT/DATA COLLECTION AND INTERVENTIONS

Nursing assessments should include the parent's knowledge base of the child's nutritional requirements, and nutritional concerns with regard to age. Nurses should provide education for the parent and child about nutritional recommendations.

Adolescence

- The rate of growth during adolescence is second only to the rate in infancy. Nutritional needs for energy, protein, calcium, iron, and zinc increase at the onset of puberty and the growth spurt.
- The female adolescent growth spurt usually begins at 10 or 11 years of age, peaks at 12 years, and is completed by 17 years. Female energy requirements are less than that of males, as they experience less growth of muscle and bone tissue and more fat deposition.
- The male adolescent growth spurt begins at 12 or 13 years of age, peaks at 14 years, and is completed by 21 years.
- Eating habits of adolescents are often inadequate in meeting recommended nutritional intake goals.

NUTRITIONAL CONSIDERATIONS

- Energy requirements average 2,000 cal/day for a 12- to 18-year-old female and 2,200 to 2,800 cal/day for a 12- to 18-year-old male.
- The USDA reports that the average U.S. adolescent consumes a diet deficient in folate, vitamins A and E, iron, zinc, magnesium, calcium, and fiber. This trend is more pronounced in females than males.
- Diets of adolescents generally exceed recommendations for total fat, saturated fat, cholesterol, sodium, and sugar.

NUTRITIONAL RISKS

Eating and snacking patterns promote essential nutrient deficiencies (calcium, vitamins, iron, fiber) and overconsumption of sugars, fat, and sodium.

- Adolescents tend to skip meals, especially breakfast, and eat more meals away from home.
- Foods are often selected from vending machines, convenience stores, and fast food restaurants. These foods are typically high in fat, sugar, and sodium.
- Carbonated beverages can replace milk and fruit juices in the diet with resulting deficiencies in vitamin C, riboflavin, phosphorous, and calcium.

Increased need for iron

- Females 14 to 18 years of age require 15 mg /day of iron to support expansion of blood volume and blood loss during menstruation.
- Males 14 to 18 years of age require 11 mg/day of iron to support expansion of muscle mass and blood volume.

Inadequate calcium intake can predispose the adolescent to osteoporosis later in life.

- During adolescence, 45% of bone mass is added.
- Normal blood-calcium levels are maintained by drawing calcium from the bones if calcium intake is low.
- Adolescents require at least 1,300 mg/day of calcium, which can be achieved by three to four servings from the dairy food group.

Dieting

- The stigma of obesity and social pressure to be thin can lead to unhealthy eating practices and poor body image, especially in females.
- Males are more susceptible to using supplements and high-protein drinks in order to build muscle mass and improve athletic performance. Some athletes restrict calories to maintain or achieve a lower weight.
- Eating disorders can follow self-imposed crash diets for weight loss.

Eating disorders (anorexia nervosa, bulimia nervosa, binge eating disorder) commonly begin during adolescence. These disorders are discussed further in the **MENTAL HEALTH REVIEW MODULE, CHAPTER 19: EATING DISORDERS**.

Adolescent pregnancy

- The physiologic demands of a growing fetus compromise the adolescent's needs for her own unfinished growth and development.
- Inconsistent eating and poor food choices place the adolescent at risk for anemia, pregnancy-induced hypertension, gestational diabetes, premature labor, miscarriage, and delivery of a newborn of low birth weight.

NURSING ASSESSMENT/DATA COLLECTION AND INTERVENTIONS

- Nursing assessments should include a determination of the following in the adolescent.
  - Typical 24-hr food intake
  - Weight patterns, current weight, and ideal body weight
  - Attitude about current weight
  - Use of nutritional supplements, vitamins, and minerals
  - Medical history and use of prescription medications
  - Use of over-the-counter medications
  - Use of substances such as marijuana, alcohol, or tobacco
  - Level of daily physical activity
- Nurses should assess for clinical findings of an eating disorder. This can include an evaluation of the adolescent's laboratory values.
- Nursing assessments should include strategies that promote health for the adolescent.
  - Educate the adolescent on using MyPlate to meet energy and nutrient needs with three regular meals and snacks.
  - Stress the importance of meeting calcium needs by including low-fat milk, yogurt, and cheese in the diet.
  - Educate the adolescent on how to select and prepare nutrient-dense snack foods: unbuttered, unsalted popcorn; pretzels; fresh fruit; string cheese; smoothies made with low-fat yogurt, skim milk, or reduced-calorie fruit juice; and raw vegetables with low-fat dips. Qpcc
  - Encourage participation in vigorous physical activity at least three times per week.
  - Refer pregnant adolescents to the Women, Infant, and Children (WIC) nutrition subsidy program.
  - Provide individual and group counseling for adolescents who have clinical findings of eating disorders.

Adulthood and older adulthood

- Nurses should assess the nutritional, physical, and mental health of adults and older adults.
- A balanced diet for all adults consists of 40% to 55% carbohydrate and 10% to 20% fat (with no more than 30% fat).
- The recommended amount for protein is unchanged in adults and older adults. However, many nutrition experts believe that protein requirements increase in older adults.
- Older adults need to reduce total caloric intake. This is due to the decrease in basal metabolic rate that occurs from the decrease in lean body mass that develops with aging. ⓖ
- Reduced caloric intake predisposes the older adult for development of nutrient deficiencies.
- Older adults can have physical, mental, and social changes that affect their ability to purchase, prepare, and digest foods and nutrients.
- Dehydration is the most common fluid and electrolyte imbalance in older adults. Fluid needs increase with medication-induced fluid losses. Some disease processes necessitate fluid restrictions.

NUTRITIONAL CONCERNS

- A 24-hr dietary intake is helpful in determining the need for dietary education.
- Older adults can have oral problems (ill-fitting dentures, difficulty chewing or swallowing), and a decrease in salivation or poor dental health. ⓖ
- Older adults have decreased cellular function and reduced body reserves, leading to decreased absorption of B_{12}, folic acid, and calcium, as well as reductions in insulin production and sensitivity.
- Decreased elasticity of blood vessels can lead to hypertension.
- Kidneys regulate the amount of potassium and sodium in the blood stream. Kidney function can decrease as much as 50% in older adults. ⓖ
- Older adults have a decreased lean muscle mass. Exercise can help to counteract muscle mass loss.
- The loss of calcium can result in decreased bone density in older adults.
- Cell-mediated immunity decreases as an individual ages.

BALANCED DIET AND NUTRIENT NEEDS

MyPlate suggests the following daily food intake for adults and older adults who get less than 30 min of moderate physical activity most days. **(7.3)**

Grains: Select whole grains.

Vegetables: Select orange and dark green leafy vegetables.

Fruits: Select fresh, dried, canned, or juices. Avoid fruits with added sugar.

> Make half your plate vegetables and fruits.

Milk, yogurt, and cheese group: One cup of milk or plain yogurt is equivalent to 1 ½ oz of natural cheese or 2 oz processed cheese.

Protein foods group: Includes meat, fish, poultry, dry beans, eggs, soy products, seeds, and nuts. One ounce-equivalent equals 1 oz meat, fish, or poultry (baked, grilled, broiled); ¼ cup cooked beans; 1 egg; 1 tbsp peanut butter; or ½ oz nuts or seeds. Use lean meats.

Oils: Use vegetable oils (except palm and coconut). One tbsp of oil equals 3 tsp equivalent; 1 tbsp mayonnaise equals 2 ½ tsp dietary intake; and 1 oz nuts equals 3 tsp oils (except hazelnut, which equals 4 tsp).

Discretionary calories: 132 to 362 discretionary calories are permitted per day. These add up quickly and can be from more than one food group.

Minerals: Calcium requirements increase for older adults as the efficiency of calcium absorption decreases with age.

Vitamins: Vitamins A, D, C, E, B_6, and B_{12} can be decreased in older adults. Supplemental vitamins are recommended. ⓖ

7.3 MyPlate recommendations for adults

	MEN			WOMEN		
	19 TO 30 YEARS	31 TO 50 YEARS	51+ YEARS	19 TO 30 YEARS	31 TO 50 YEARS	51+ YEARS
Calories	2,400	2,200	2,000	2,000	1,800	1,600
Fruits	2 cups	2 cups	2 cups	2 cups	1 ½ cups	1 ½ cups
Vegetables	3 cups	3 cups	2 ½ cups	2 ½ cups	2 ½ cups	2 cups
Grains	8 oz	7 oz	6 oz	6 oz	6 oz	5 oz
Protein	6 ½ oz-eq	6 oz-eq	5 ½ oz-eq	5 ½ oz-eq	5 oz-eq	5 oz-eq
Milk	3 cups	3 cups	3 cups	3 cups	3 cups	3 cups
Oils	7 tsp	6 tsp	6 tsp	6 tsp	5 tsp	5 tsp

Source: United States Department of Agriculture. ChooseMyPlate.gov. Retrieved December 22, 2015, from www.choosemyplate.gov

REGULAR EXERCISE

- All adults should exercise at a moderate or vigorous pace for at least 30 min/day, 3 to 7 days/week.
- Physical activity must increase heart rate to be relevant. Moderate activities include gardening/yard work, golf, dancing, and walking briskly.
- The loss of lean muscle mass is part of normal aging and can be decreased with regular exercise. The loss of lean muscle can be associated with a decrease in total protein and insulin sensitivity.
- Regular exercise can improve bone density, relieve depression, and enhance cardiovascular and respiratory function.

POTENTIAL EFFECT OF PHYSICAL, MENTAL, AND SOCIAL CHANGES

- Diseases and treatments can interfere with nutrient and food absorption, and utilization.
  - Aging adults are at an increased risk for developing osteoporosis (decreasing total bone mass and deterioration of bone tissue). Adequate calcium and vitamin D intake with regular weight-bearing exercise is important for maximizing bone density. ©
  - Osteoarthritis (OA) causes significant disability and pain in older adult clients. OA can limit mobility and present difficulty in obtaining and preparing proper foods.
  - Arthritis can interfere with the purchase and preparation of foods.
  - Alzheimer's disease is a form of dementia commonly seen in clients age 65 and older. This form of dementia causes impairments in memory and judgment that can make shopping, storing, and cooking food difficult.
- Some medications (diuretics) for hypertension can cause sodium or potassium losses.
- Loss of smell and vision interfere with the interest in eating food.
- BMI should be between 18.5 and 24.9. There is an increased risk for both overweight and underweight older adult clients. Overweight adults are more prone to hypertension, diabetes mellitus, and stroke.
- Older adults can have difficulty chewing, in which case mincing or chopping food is helpful. They can have difficulty swallowing food, and thickened liquids can decrease the risk for aspiration.
- Social isolation, loss of a partner, and mental deterioration can cause poor nutrition in adult and older adult clients. Encourage socialization and refer to a senior center or program. Qpcc
- A fixed income can make it difficult for older adults to purchase needed foods. Refer to food programs, senior centers, and food banks. Meals on Wheels programs are available for housebound older adults.

FLUID INTAKE

- The long-held standard of consuming eight 8-oz glasses of liquid per day has been tempered by evidence that dehydration is not imminent even when less than 64 oz of fluid is consumed.
- Solid foods provide varying amounts of water, making it possible to get adequate fluid despite low beverage intake.
- For healthy adults, it is generally acceptable to allow normal drinking and eating habits to provide needed fluids.
- Encourage water and natural juices, and discourage drinking only soda pop and other liquids that have caffeine.

NURSING ASSESSMENT/DATA COLLECTION AND INTERVENTIONS

- Nursing assessments should include a dietary profile of the adult or older adult. Medical history, medication regimen, mobility, social practices, mental status, and financial circumstances are important components of the assessment.
- Nurses should provide education about proper dietary practices for the adult and older adult, while additionally providing referrals to community agencies when appropriate.

Application Exercises

1. A nurse in an assisted living facility is caring for an older adult client. The nurse should recognize that older adults have decreased absorption of which of the following? (Select all that apply.)
   A. Calcium
   B. Chloride
   C. Folic acid
   D. Magnesium
   E. Phosphorus

2. A nurse is assessing a 6-month-old infant who has a lactose intolerance. Which of the following findings should the nurse expect? (Select all that apply.)
   A. Abdominal distention
   B. Flatus
   C. Hypoactive bowel sounds
   D. Occasional diarrhea
   E. Visible peristalsis

3. A nurse is educating the parents of a toddler about appropriate snack foods. Which of the following foods should the nurse include in the teaching? (Select all that apply.)
   A. Graham crackers
   B. Apple slices
   C. Raisins
   D. Jelly beans
   E. Cheese cubes

4. A nurse is teaching a group of pregnant clients about iron-rich foods. Which of the following foods should the nurse include in the teaching? (Select all that apply.)
   A. Beans
   B. Fish
   C. Dairy products
   D. Lean red meats
   E. Apples

5. A school nurse is teaching a group of teens about healthy snack food choices. Which of the following foods should the nurse include in the teaching? (Select all that apply.)
   A. Carrot sticks with low-fat dip
   B. Cheese and crackers
   C. Unbuttered popcorn
   D. French fries
   E. Hot dog

PRACTICE Active Learning Scenario

A community health nurse is teaching a group of parents the importance of adequate vitamin D intake for children. Use the ATI Active Learning Template: Basic Concept to complete this item.

UNDERLYING PRINCIPLES
- Explain why vitamin D is important for children.
- Identify at least two sources of vitamin D.

Application Exercises Key

1. A. **CORRECT:** Older adults have decreased cellular function and reduced body reserves, leading to decreased absorption of B_{12}, folic acid, and calcium.

   B. Older adults do not have decreased absorption of chloride.

   C. **CORRECT:** Older adults have decreased cellular function and reduced body reserves, leading to decreased absorption of B_{12}, folic acid, and calcium.

   D. Older adults do not have decreased absorption of magnesium.

   E. Older adults do not have decreased absorption of phosphorus.

   Ⓝ *NCLEX® Connection: Health Promotion and Maintenance, Health Promotion/Disease Prevention*

2. A. **CORRECT:** Abdominal distention is a clinical finding associated with a lactose intolerance.

   B. **CORRECT:** Flatus is a clinical finding associated with a lactose intolerance.

   C. Hypoactive bowel sounds are not associated with a lactose intolerance.

   D. **CORRECT:** Occasional diarrhea is a clinical finding associated with a lactose intolerance.

   E. Visible peristalsis is not associated with a lactose intolerance.

   Ⓝ *NCLEX® Connection: Health Promotion and Maintenance, Aging Process*

3. A. **CORRECT:** Graham crackers are appropriate snack foods for toddlers.

   B. **CORRECT:** Apple slices are appropriate snack foods for toddlers.

   C. Raisins are difficult to chew and pose a choking hazard.

   D. Jelly beans are difficult to swallow, pose a choking risk, and are high in sugar content.

   E. **CORRECT:** Cheese cubes are appropriate snack foods for toddlers.

   Ⓝ *NCLEX® Connection: Health Promotion and Maintenance, Aging Process*

4. A. **CORRECT:** Iron-rich foods include beans.

   B. **CORRECT:** Iron-rich foods include fish.

   C. **CORRECT:** Iron-rich foods include dairy products.

   D. **CORRECT:** Iron-rich foods include lean red meats.

   E. Apples are not rich in iron.

   Ⓝ *NCLEX® Connection: Health Promotion and Maintenance, Ante/Intra/Postpartum and Newborn Care*

5. A. **CORRECT:** Carrot sticks with low-fat ranch dip are a healthy snack selection.

   B. **CORRECT:** Cheese and crackers are a healthy snack selection.

   C. **CORRECT:** Unbuttered popcorn is a healthy snack selection.

   D. French fries are not a healthy food choice because they are high in fat.

   E. Hot dogs are not a healthy food choice because they are high in sodium and fat.

   Ⓝ *NCLEX® Connection: Health Promotion and Maintenance, Aging Process*

PRACTICE Answer

Using the ATI Active Learning Template: Basic Concept

UNDERLYING PRINCIPLES

- Vitamin D is essential for the development of healthy bones. It is important in children because their bones are newly formed and continually growing.
- Vitamin D aids in the absorption of calcium into the bones. Sunlight exposure, milk (cow's, soy), and fatty fish are sources of vitamin D.

Ⓝ *NCLEX® Connection: Health Promotion and Maintenance, Aging Process*

When reviewing the following chapters, keep in mind the relevant topics and tasks of the NCLEX outline, in particular:

Client Needs: Basic Care and Comfort

NUTRITION AND ORAL HYDRATION
Manage the client's nutritional intake.

Provide client nutrition through continuous or intermittent tube feedings.

Evaluate side effects of client tube feedings and intervene, as needed.

Client Needs: Reduction of Risk Potential

LABORATORY VALUES: Compare client laboratory values to normal laboratory values.

POTENTIAL FOR ALTERATIONS IN BODY SYSTEMS:
Identify client potential for skin breakdown.

UNIT 2   CLINICAL NUTRITION

CHAPTER 8 *Modified Diets*

Therapeutic nutrition is the role of food and nutrition in the treatment of diseases and disorders. The basic diet becomes therapeutic when modifications are made to meet client needs. Modifications can include increasing or decreasing caloric intake, fiber, or other specific nutrients; omitting specific foods; and modifying the consistency of foods.

It is important to remember, however, that food meets both physiological and psychological needs and should be a pleasant experience for the hospitalized client. Nurses should collaborate with the dietitian for nutritional or dietary concerns. Q℡

TYPES OF THERAPEUTIC DIETS

Clear liquid diet

- Consists of foods or fluids that have no residue and are liquid at room temperature.
- Primarily to prevent dehydration and relieve thirst, the diet consists of water and carbohydrates. This diet requires minimal digestion, leaves minimal residue, and is non-gas-forming. It is nutritionally inadequate and should not be used long-term.
- Indications include acute illness, reduction of colon fecal material prior to certain diagnostic tests and procedures, acute gastrointestinal disorders, and some postoperative recovery.
- Acceptable foods are water, tea, coffee, fat-free broth, carbonated beverages, clear juices, ginger ale, and gelatin.
- Limit caffeine consumption, which can lead to increased hydrochloric acid and upset stomach.

Full liquid diet

- Consists of foods that are liquid at room temperature.
- Offers more variety and nutritional support than a clear liquid diet and can supply adequate amounts of energy and nutrients.
- Acceptable foods include all liquids on a clear liquid diet, all forms of milk, soups, vegetable and fruit juices, eggnog, plain ice cream and sherbet, refined or strained cereals, and puddings.
- Evaluate the need for high-protein and high-calorie supplements if this diet is used more than 2 to 3 days.
- Indications include a transition from liquid to soft diets, postoperative recovery, acute gastritis, febrile conditions, and intolerance of solid foods.
- Provides oral nourishment for clients having difficulty chewing or swallowing solid foods. Use cautiously with clients who have dysphagia (difficulty swallowing) unless liquids are thickened appropriately. Qs
- Contraindicated for clients who have lactose intolerance or hypercholesterolemia. Use lactose-reduced milk and dairy products when possible.

Blenderized liquid (pureed) diet

- Consists of liquids and foods that are pureed to liquid form.
- The composition and consistency of a pureed diet varies, depending on the client's needs.
- Modify with regard to calories, protein, fat, or other nutrients based on the dietary needs of the client. Qᴘᴄᴄ
- Adding broth, milk, gravy, cream, soup, tomato sauce, or fruit juice to foods in place of water provides additional calories and nutritional value.
- Each food is pureed separately to preserve individual flavor.
- Indications include clients who have chewing or swallowing difficulties, oral or facial surgery, and wired jaws.

Soft (bland, low-fiber) diet

- Contains whole foods that are low in fiber, lightly seasoned, and easily digested.
- Food supplements or snacks in between meals add calories.
- Food selections vary and can include smooth, creamy, or crisp textures. Raw fruits and vegetables, coarse breads and cereals, beans, and other potentially gas-forming foods are excluded.
- Indications include clients transitioning between full liquid and regular diets, and those who have acute infections, chewing difficulties, or gastrointestinal disorders.
- Predisposes clients to constipation.

Mechanical soft diet

- A regular diet that is modified in texture. The diet composition is altered for specific nutrient needs.
- Includes foods that require minimal chewing before swallowing (ground meats, canned fruits, softly cooked vegetables).
- Butter, gravies, sugar, or honey may be added to increase calorie intake.
- Excludes harder foods (dried fruits, most raw fruits and vegetables, foods containing seeds and nuts).
- Indications include limited chewing ability; dysphagia, poorly fitting dentures, and clients who are edentulous (without teeth); surgery to the head, neck, or mouth; and strictures of the intestinal tract.

Dysphagia diet

- Prescribed when swallowing is impaired, such as following a stroke.
- Signs of dysphagia are drooling, pocketing food, choking, or gagging.

LEVELS OF SOLID TEXTURES

- **Level 1: Pureed.** Foods are totally pureed to a smooth consistency with a pudding-like texture (pureed fruits, vegetables, meats, soups, scrambled eggs, pudding, custard, applesauce).
- **Level 2: Mechanically altered.** Soft-textured, moist, semi-solid foods that are easily chewed and swallowed (ground meat served with gravy, chicken or tuna salad, well-moistened pancakes with syrup, poached eggs, soft canned or cooked fruit).
- **Level 3: Advanced.** Near-normal textured foods that are moist (moist tender meats or casseroles, breads that are not crusty, moist potatoes, soups, rice and stuffing). Hard, sticky foods are eliminated.

LEVELS OF LIQUID CONSISTENCIES

- **Thin:** Non-restrictive. Consists of all unthickened beverages and supplements (clear juices, frozen yogurt, ice cream, milk, soda and broth).
- **Nectar-like:** Consists of liquids that are thin enough to sip through a straw but thicker than water. Consistency of a heavy syrup (nectars, cream soups, buttermilk and thin milkshakes).
- **Honey-like:** Liquids are pourable but thickened. They can be eaten with a spoon but cannot be sipped through a straw (honey, tomato sauce and yogurt).
- **Spoon-thick:** Consists of liquids thickened to maintain their shape and need to be eaten with a spoon (pudding, custard, hot cereals).

Regular diet (normal or house diet)

- Indicated for clients who do not need dietary restrictions. The diet is adjusted to meet age specific needs throughout the life cycle.
- Many health care facilities offer self-select menus for regular diets.
- Modify the regular diet to accommodate individual preferences, food habits, and ethnic values. Qᴘᴄᴄ

NURSING ASSESSMENT/DATA COLLECTION AND INTERVENTIONS

- Ongoing assessment parameters include daily weights, prescribed laboratory tests, and an evaluation of a client's nutritional and energy needs and response to diet therapy.
- Observe and document nutritional intake. Perform a calorie count if needed to determine caloric intake and to evaluate adequacy.
- Provide education and support for diet therapy.
- A prescription for a diet as tolerated permits a client's preferences while taking into consideration the client's ability to eat. Assess the client for hunger, appetite, and nausea when planning the most appropriate diet, and consult with a dietitian.
- Dietary intake is progressively increased (from nothing by mouth to clear liquids to regular diet) following a major surgery. Nurses should assess for the return of bowel function (as evidenced by auscultation of bowel sounds and the passage of flatus) before advancing a client's diet. Qᴇʙᴘ

Application Exercises

1. A nurse is caring for a client following an appendectomy. The nurse verifies the postoperative prescription, which reads "discontinue NPO status; advance diet as tolerated." Which of the following are appropriate for the nurse to offer the client? (Select all that apply.)

   A. Applesauce

   B. Chicken broth

   C. Sherbet

   D. Wheat toast

   E. Cranberry juice

2. A nurse is caring for a client who is to receive a Level 2 dysphagia diet due to a recent stroke. Which of the following dietary selections is most appropriate?

   A. Turkey sandwich

   B. Poached eggs

   C. Peanut butter crackers

   D. Granola

3. A nurse is performing dietary needs assessments for a group of clients. A blenderized liquid diet is appropriate for which of the following clients? (Select all that apply.)

   A. A client who has a wired jaw due to a motor vehicle crash

   B. A client who is 24 hr postoperative following temporomandibular joint repair

   C. A client who has difficulty chewing due to oral surgery

   D. A client who has hypercholesterolemia due to coronary artery disease

   E. A client who is scheduled for a colonoscopy the next morning

4. A nurse is caring for a client who has multiple sclerosis and requires liquids with honey-like thickness. Which of the following foods can the client consume without adding a thickening agent?

   A. Ice cream

   B. Yogurt

   C. Buttermilk

   D. Cream of chicken soup

5. A nurse is assisting a client who has a prescription for a mechanical soft diet with food selections. Which of the following are appropriate selections by the client? (Select all that apply.)

   A. Dried prunes

   B. Ground turkey

   C. Mashed carrots

   D. Fresh strawberries

   E. Cottage cheese

PRACTICE Active Learning Scenario

A nurse is planning care for a client who is to receive a full liquid diet due to an acute gastrointestinal infection. Use the ATI Active Learning Template: Basic Concept to complete this item to include the following sections:

UNDERLYING PRINCIPLES: Identify the indication for a regular diet.

NURSING INTERVENTIONS:

- Identify at least two assessments that are appropriate to determine the need for dietary modifications to the regular diet.
- Identify at least two nursing actions that are appropriate to monitor the client's response to diet therapy.

1. A. Applesauce is appropriate once the client's diet begins to advance. It is not appropriate as an initial postoperative selection.

    B. **CORRECT:** Chicken broth is a clear liquid, which is appropriate as an initial selection for a client who is postoperative.

    C. Sherbet is appropriate once the client's diet begins to advance. It is not appropriate as an initial postoperative selection.

    D. Wheat toast is appropriate once the client's diet begins to advance. It is not appropriate as an initial postoperative selection.

    E. **CORRECT:** Cranberry juice is a clear liquid, which is appropriate as an initial selection for a client who is postoperative.

    Ⓝ *NCLEX® Connection: Basic Care and Comfort, Nutrition and Oral Hydration*

2. A. A Level 2 diet requires foods that are moist and semi-solid. A turkey sandwich would be too dry, and breads are not allowed on the Level 2 diet. This would be an appropriate choice for a client receiving a regular diet.

    B. **CORRECT:** A Level 2 diet requires foods that are moist and semi-solid, such as a poached egg.

    C. A Level 2 diet requires foods that are moist and semi-solid. Peanut butter crackers are too sticky and dry for a Level 2 diet. This would be an appropriate choice for a client who is receiving a regular diet.

    D. A Level 2 diet requires foods that are moist and semi-solid. Granola is too hard and crunchy for a client receiving a Level 2 diet.

    Ⓝ *NCLEX® Connection: Reduction of Risk Potential, Potential for Complications of Diagnostic Tests/Treatments/Procedures*

3. A. **CORRECT:** A blenderized liquid diet is appropriate for a client who has a wired jaw.

    B. **CORRECT:** A blenderized liquid diet is appropriate for a client following oral surgery.

    C. **CORRECT:** A blenderized liquid diet is appropriate for a client who has difficulty chewing.

    D. The client's history does not indicate a need for a blenderized liquid diet.

    E. A client who is scheduled for a colonoscopy should receive a clear liquid, rather than a blenderized liquid, diet.

    Ⓝ *NCLEX® Connection: Reduction of Risk Potential, Potential for Alterations in Body Systems*

4. A. The nurse should identify ice cream as a thin liquid that can place the client at risk for aspiration.

    B. **CORRECT:** The nurse should identify yogurt as a honey-like liquid, because it can be eaten with a spoon but not sipped with a straw. This client can also safely receive spoon-thick liquids.

    C. The nurse should identify buttermilk as a nectar-like liquid that can place the client at risk for aspiration.

    D. The nurse should identify cream of chicken soup as a nectar-like liquid that can place the client at risk for aspiration.

    Ⓝ *NCLEX® Connection: Basic Care and Comfort, Nutrition and Oral Hydration*

5. A. Dried fruits are excluded from a mechanical soft diet due to potential chewing difficulty.

    B. **CORRECT:** Ground meats require minimal chewing before swallowing and are therefore appropriate for a mechanical soft diet.

    C. **CORRECT:** Mashed carrots require minimal chewing before swallowing and are therefore appropriate for a mechanical soft diet.

    D. Fresh strawberries are excluded from a mechanical soft diet due to seeds and potential chewing difficulty.

    E. **CORRECT:** Cottage cheese requires minimal chewing before swallowing and is therefore appropriate for a mechanical soft diet.

    Ⓝ *NCLEX® Connection: Basic Care and Comfort, Nutrition and Oral Hydration*

PRACTICE Answer

Using the ATI Active Learning Template: Basic Concept

UNDERLYING PRINCIPLES: A regular diet is indicated for clients who do not need dietary restrictions.

NURSING INTERVENTIONS
Assessments to determine the need for dietary modification
• Individual preferences.
• Food habits.
• Ethnic values or practices.
Assessments to monitor the client's response to diet therapy
• Obtain daily weight.
• Monitor laboratory values.
• Monitor energy level.
• Observe and document nutritional intake.
• Evaluate understanding of diet therapy.

Ⓝ *NCLEX® Connection: Physiological Adaptation, Illness Management*

UNIT 2   CLINICAL NUTRITION

CHAPTER 9 *Enteral Nutrition*

Enteral nutrition (EN) is used when a client cannot consume adequate nutrients and calories orally, but maintains a partially functional gastrointestinal (GI) system. EN is contraindicated when the GI tract is nonfunctional, such as in the cases of paralytic ileus or intestinal obstruction.

EN is administered when a client has a medical condition (burns, trauma, radiation therapy or chemotherapy, liver or renal dysfunction, infection and inflammatory bowel disease) that hinders the client's nutritional status. EN is also administered when a client is neuromuscularly impaired and cannot chew or swallow food.

EN feeding or gavage feeding for an infant is used when an infant is too weak for sucking, unable to coordinate swallowing, and lacks a gag reflex. Gavage feeding is implemented to conserve energy when an infant is attempting to breast feed or bottle feed, but becomes fatigued, weak, or cyanotic.

EN consists of a commercial formula administered by a tube into the stomach or small intestine. Enteral feedings most closely utilize the body's own digestive and metabolic routes. EN can augment an oral diet or be the sole source of nutrition.

ENTERAL FEEDING ROUTES

A client's medical status and the anticipated length of time that a tube feeding will be required determine the type of tube used.

Nasoenteric tubes

Nasoenteric tubes are short-term (less than 3 to 4 weeks).
- **Nasogastric** (NG) tubes are passed through the nose to the stomach.
- **Nasoduodenal** tubes pass from the nose through the stomach and end in the duodenum.
- **Nasojejunal** tubes pass from the nose through the stomach and end in the jejunum.
- Nasoduodenal and nasojejunal tubes are used in clients who are at risk for aspiration or who have delayed gastric emptying (gastroparesis).
- For an infant, a feeding tube is inserted from the nares or mouth into the stomach. This flexible tube can remain taped in place for up to 30 days.

Ostomies

Ostomies are placed for clients requiring long-term enteral feeding, who are at high risk for aspiration or when a nasal obstruction makes insertion through the nose impossible. An ostomy is a surgically created opening (stoma) made to deliver feedings directly into the stomach or intestines.

Gastrostomy tubes are endoscopically or surgically inserted into the stomach.
- A percutaneous endoscopic gastrostomy (PEG) tube is placed with the aid of an endoscope.
- An alternative to the PEG tube is a skin-level gastrostomy tube, which is known as a low-profile gastrostomy device. It is more comfortable, longer-lasting, and fully immersible in water. Checking for residual is more difficult with this device because of the close proximity of the button on the skin.
- Gastrostomy tube feedings are generally well-tolerated because the stomach chamber holds and releases feedings in a physiologic manner that promotes effective digestion. As a result, dumping syndrome is usually avoided.

Jejunostomy tubes are surgically inserted into the jejunal portion of the small intestine (jejunum).

ENTERAL FEEDING FORMULAS

- Commercial products are preferred over home-blended ingredients because the nutrient composition, consistency and safety can be better insured.
- Standard and hydrolyzed formulas are the two primary types of enteral feeding formulas available. They are categorized by the complexity of the proteins included.

Standard formulas

- Also called polymeric or intact, are composed of whole proteins (milk, meat, eggs) or protein isolates.
- These formulas require a functioning gastrointestinal tract.
- Most provide 1.0 to 1.2 cal/mL, but are available in high-protein, high-calorie, fiber-enriched, and disease-specific formulas.

Hydrolyzed formulas

- Also called elemental, these are composed of partially digested protein peptides and free amino acids.
- These formulas are used for clients who have a partially functioning gastrointestinal tract, or those who have an impaired ability to digest and absorb foods (inflammatory bowel disease, liver failure, cystic fibrosis, pancreatic disorders, and for clients who have an impaired immune system).
- Most provide 1.0 to 1.5 cal/mL. High-calorie formulas provide 1.5 to 2.0 cal/mL. Partially hydrolyzed formulas provide other nutrients in simpler forms that require little or no digestion.

PACKAGING

Tube feedings can be packaged in cans or prefilled bags.
- Prefilled bags and administration tubing should be discarded every 24 hr or according to facility policy, even if they are not empty.
- Cans can be used to add formula to a generic bag to infuse via a pump, or for feedings directly from a syringe.

DETERMINING APPROPRIATE FORMULA

Caloric density determines the volume of the formula necessary to meet the caloric needs of a client (1.0 to 1.2 cal/mL).

Water content in formulas with 1.0 cal/mL should be 850 mL water per 1 L formula. Higher-calorie formulas have lower water content. The client can need additional free water to meet hydration needs.

Osmolality of the formula is determined by the concentration of sugars, amino acids, and electrolytes.
- Osmolality is increased if the formula contains more digested protein.
- Hydrolyzed or partially hydrolyzed (predigested) formulas are higher in osmolality than standard formulas. They are also lactose-free.

Fiber and residue content
- Standard formulas are low in residue which makes them less likely to produce abdominal distention or gas. These products are optimal for clients who have been on bowel rest, are postoperative following bowel surgery, or have GI related disease processes. Hydrolyzed formulas are considered residual free.
- Standard formulas that are enriched with fiber are recommended for clients who have constipation or diarrhea to normalize bowel movements.

The presence of **other nutrients** include fats and carbohydrates, which can be modified according to a client's disease processes (respiratory disease, malabsorption, diabetes mellitus, kidney disease).

ENTERAL FEEDING DELIVERY METHODS

The delivery method is dependent on the type and location of the feeding tube, type of formula administered, and the client's medical status and GI function.

Continuous infusion method

Formula is administered at a continuous rate over a 12- to 24-hr period.
- Infusion pumps help ensure consistent flow rates.
- This method is recommended for critically ill clients because of its association with smaller residual volumes, and a lower risk of aspiration and diarrhea.
- Residual volumes should be measured every 4 to 6 hr.
- Feeding tubes should be flushed with water every 4 hr to maintain tube patency and provide hydration.
- If the client's gastric residual volume exceeds 250 mL for each of two consecutive assessments or the amount stated in hospital policy or provider's prescription, the continuous feeding should be held and the client's tolerance should be re-assessed. In children, residual volumes should be measured and feedings held if the amount is equal to or greater than ¼ the prescribed feeding amount. The residual should be returned and then the amount rechecked in 30 min. to 1 hr.

Cyclic feeding

- Formula is administered at a continuous rate over an 8- to 12-hr time period, often during sleeping hours.
- Often used for transition from total EN to oral intake.

Intermittent tube feeding

Formula is administered every 4 to 6 hr in equal portions of 250 to 400 mL over a 30- to 60-min time frame, usually by gravity drip or an electronic pump.
- Often used for noncritical clients, home tube feedings, and clients in rehabilitation.
- Resembles normal pattern of nutrient intake.
- Residual volumes should be measured prior to initiating the feeding and held if the amount is greater than the amount stated in hospital policy or prescription.

Bolus feeding

A variation of intermittent feeding using a large syringe attached to the feeding tube. A large volume of formula (700 mL maximum, usual volume is 250 to 400 mL) is administered over a short period of time, usually in 15 to 30 min, four to six times daily.
- The rate of administration for a premature or small infant should be no greater than 5 mL every 10 min, and 10 mL/min in older infants and children.
- Bolus feedings are delivered directly into the stomach; they are contraindicated for tubes placed into the jejunum or duodenum. They can be poorly tolerated and can cause dumping syndrome.

NURSING ACTIONS

PREPARATION OF THE CLIENT

- Prior to instilling enteral feeding, tube placement should be verified by radiography. The tube should then be marked with indelible ink or adhesive tape where it exits the nose and documented. The tube should be measured each shift and prior to each feeding to ensure the tube has not migrated. Aspirating gastric contents and measuring pH levels are not considered reliable methods of verifying initial placement. Q**EBP**
- Verify the presence of bowel sounds.
- To maintain feeding tube patency, it is flushed routinely with warm water.
  - Gastric residuals should be checked every 4 to 6 hr. If the residual volume exceeds current residual guidelines, facility policy, or provider prescription, it can be necessary to consider reducing the rate of the feeding. Residuals should be returned to the stomach as they contain electrolytes, nutrients, and digestive enzymes. Follow facility policy.
  - **FOR AN INFANT:** Subtract the amount of the residual from the amount of the formula to be given. Return the residual to the stomach plus the reduced amount of formula or breast milk.
  - **FOR CHILDREN:** If the residual is more than one fourth of the previous feeding, return the residual to the stomach, hold the feeding, and recheck in 30 to 60 min.
  - Notify the provider if a large amount of residual continues to occur.
- The head of the bed should be elevated at least 30° during feedings and for at least 30 to 60 min afterward to lessen the risk of aspiration. Q**s**
- Burp the infant following the feeding if the infant's condition allows.
- Begin with a small volume of full-strength formula. Increase volume in intervals as tolerated until the desired volume is achieved.
- Administer the feeding solution at room temperature to decrease gastrointestinal discomfort.
- Do not heat formulas in a microwave as this can result in uneven temperatures within the solution.

BASELINE PARAMETERS
- Obtain height, weight, and body mass index.
- Monitor serum albumin, hemoglobin, hematocrit, glucose, blood urea nitrogen (BUN), and electrolyte levels.
- Evaluate the client's nutritional and energy needs.
- Verify gastrointestinal function. Dysfunction of the gastrointestinal tract can indicate a need for alternate forms of nutrition.

ONGOING CARE

- Monitor daily weights and I&O.
- Obtain gastric residuals every 4 to 6 hr.
- Monitor electrolytes, BUN, creatinine, serum minerals, and CBC.
- Monitor the tube site for manifestations of infection or intolerance (pain, redness, swelling, drainage).
- Monitor the character and frequency of bowel movements.
- When appropriate, administer medications through a feeding tube.
  - Feeding should be stopped prior to administering medications.
  - The tubing should be flushed with water (15 to 30 mL) before and after the medication is administered, and between each medication if more than one is administered.
  - Medications should only be dissolved in water.
  - Liquid medications should be used when possible.
    - For an infant or child, the volume of water to flush is 1.5 times the amount predetermined to flush an unused feeding tube of the same size.
    - More water can be required to flush the tubing following some medications (suspensions).

INTERVENTIONS

- Weaning occurs as oral consumption increases. Enteral feedings can be discontinued when the client consumes two-thirds of protein and calorie needs orally for 3 to 5 days.
- A client who is NPO will require meticulous oral care.
- A client can require nutritional support service at home for long-term EN. A interprofessional team comprised of a nurse, dietitian, pharmacist, and the provider monitors the client's weight, electrolyte balance, and overall physical condition. Q**TC**
- Transitioning from EN to an oral diet requires the client to receive adequate nutrition as food items are reintroduced.
  - Begin the transition process by stopping the EN for 1 hr before a meal.
  - Slowly increase the frequency of the meals until the client is eating six small meals daily.
  - When oral intake equals 500 to 750 cal/day, the continuous tube feeding is administered only during the night.

COMPLICATIONS

Gastrointestinal complications

- Constipation, diarrhea, cramping, pain, abdominal distention, dumping syndrome, nausea, and vomiting.
- Dumping syndrome occurs due to rapid emptying of the formula into the small intestine, resulting in a fluid shift. Manifestations include dizziness, rapid pulse, diaphoresis, pallor, and lightheadedness.

NURSING ACTIONS

- Consider a change in formula.
- Decrease the flow rate or total volume of the infusion.
- Increase the volume of free water if constipated.
- Administer the EN at room temperature.
- Take measures to prevent bacterial contamination.

Mechanical complications

Tube misplacement or dislodgement; aspiration; irritation and leakage at the insertion site; irritation of the nose, esophagus, and mucosa; and clogging of the feeding tube.

NURSING ACTIONS

- Confirm tube placement prior to feedings
- Elevate the head of the bed at least 30° during feedings and maintain client in this position for approximately 60 min following completion of the feeding.
- Administer bolus feedings over a period of 15 to 30 min.
- Monitor gastric residuals and hold feedings per prescription or hospital policy.
- Flush the tubing with 15 to 30 mL of warm water every 4 hr for continuous infusion, after returning residual formula into the stomach, and before and after bolus feedings, and between each medication administration.
- Unclog tubing using gentle pressure with 30 to 50 mL warm water in a 60 mL piston syringe. Use carbonated beverages only when water does not open the tubing. Commercially made products are also available and have been shown to effectively dissolve clotted formula.
- Do not mix medications with the formula.

Metabolic complications

Include dehydration, hyperglycemia, electrolyte imbalances, fluid overload, refeeding syndrome, or rapid weight gain.

NURSING ACTIONS

- Provide adequate amounts of free water.
- Consider changing formula to one that is isotonic.
- Restrict fluids if fluid overload occurs.
- Monitor electrolytes, serum glucose, and weights.
- Monitor respiratory, cardiovascular and neurological status.
- Administer insulin per prescribed protocol for hyperglycemia.

Refeeding syndrome

A potentially fatal complication that occurs when a client who is in a starvation state is started on enteral nutrition. This occurs because of electrolyte shifts and altered glucose levels once feeding restarts.

NURSING ACTIONS

- Monitor the client for changes in respiratory, neurological, and cardiac status, promptly notifying the provider if they occur.
- Monitor serum electrolyte levels.

Food poisoning

Can result due to bacterial contamination of formula.

NURSING ACTIONS: Prevent bacterial contamination.
- Wash hands before handling formula or enteral products.
- Clean equipment and tops of formula cans.
- Used closed feeding systems
- Cover and label unused cans with the client's name, room number, date, and time of opening.
- Refrigerate unused portions promptly for up to 24 hr.
- Replace the feeding bag, administration tubing, and any equipment used to mix the formula every 24 hr.
- Fill generic bags with only 4 hr worth of formula.

Application Exercises

1. A nurse is discussing the use of a low-profile gastrostomy device with the parent of a child who is receiving an enteral feeding. Which of the following is an appropriate statement by the nurse?

   A. "The device can be uncomfortable for children."

   B. "Checking residual is much easier with this device."

   C. "Tub baths are allowed with this device."

   D. "Mobility of the child is limited with this device."

2. A nurse is teaching a client who is starting continuous feedings about the various types of enteral nutrition (EN) formulas. Which of the following should the nurse include in the teaching?

   A. Formula rich in fiber is recommended when starting EN.

   B. Standard formula contains whole protein.

   C. Hydrolyzed formula is recommended for a full-functioning GI tract.

   D. The high-calorie formula has increased water content.

3. A nurse is planning care for a client who is receiving enteral nutrition through continuous infusion. Which of the following interventions should be included in the plan of care? (Select all that apply.)

   A. Administer with an infusion pump.

   B. Measure residual every 8 hr.

   C. Flush the feeding tube every 4 hr.

   D. Reinstill the residual feeding into the stomach.

   E. Reassess tolerance if the residual volume is greater than the prescribed amount.

4. A nurse is administering bolus enteral feedings to a client who has malnutrition. Which of the following are appropriate nursing interventions? (Select all that apply.)

   A. Verify the presence of bowel sounds.

   B. Flush the feeding tube with warm water.

   C. Elevate the head of the bed 20°.

   D. Administer the feeding at room temperature.

   E. Inspect the tube insertion site.

5. A nurse is preparing to administer intermittent enteral feeding to a client who has neuromuscular disorder. Which of the following are appropriate nursing interventions? (Select all that apply.)

   A. Fill the feeding bag with 24 hr worth of formula.

   B. Discard feeding equipment after 24 hr.

   C. Leave unused portions of formula at the bedside.

   D. Label the unused portion of the formula.

   E. Elevate the head of the client's bed for 15 min after administration.

PRACTICE Active Learning Scenario

A nurse is providing information to a client on complications that can occur when administering an enteral nutrition. What information should the nurse include in the teaching? Use the ATI Active Learning Template: Basic Concept to complete this item to include the following.

RELATED CONTENT: Identify three complications. List two nursing interventions for each complication.

Application Exercises Key

1. A. The gastrostomy device is more comfortable for children because of the close proximity of the button on the skin.

   B. Checking for residual is more difficult with this device because of the close proximity of the button on the skin.

   C. **CORRECT:** The low-profile gastrostomy device is fully immersible in water.

   D. The mobility of the child is increased because of the close proximity of the button on the skin.

   (N) *NCLEX® Connection: Basic Care and Comfort, Nutrition and Oral Hydration*

2. A. Residual-free formula without fiber is recommended when starting EN to minimize abdominal distention from increased flatus.

   B. **CORRECT:** A standard formula contains whole protein (milk, meat, eggs) and requires a full-functioning GI tract.

   C. Hydrolyzed formula is recommended for a partially functioning digestive tract or for those who have impaired ability to digest and absorb foods.

   D. Formula high in calories is low in water content.

   (N) *NCLEX® Connection: Basic Care and Comfort, Nutrition and Oral Hydration*

3. A. **CORRECT:** Administering continuous drip enteral nutrition using an infusion pump ensures the correct volume of the feeding is being infused.

   B. The measurement of residual is performed every 4 to 6 hr to determine if the formula is being digested.

   C. **CORRECT:** Flushing the feeding tube every 4 hr maintains patency.

   D. **CORRECT:** Reinstilling the residual feeding into the stomach returns needed fluids, electrolytes, nutrients, and digestive enzymes.

   E. **CORRECT:** The client's tolerance of the amount and type of formula used should be reassessed if the residual volume is greater than the prescribed amount as this is an indication that the amounts infused are not being digested.

   (N) *NCLEX® Connection: Basic Care and Comfort, Nutrition and Oral Hydration*

4. A. **CORRECT:** The nurse should verify the presence of bowel sounds prior to a bolus feeding to ensure the bowel is functioning.

   B. **CORRECT:** The nurse should flush the feeding tube to ensure patency before administering a bolus feeding.

   C. The nurse should elevate the client's head of bed at least 30° prior to a bolus feeding to decrease the risk of aspiration.

   D. **CORRECT:** The nurse should administer the bolus feeding at room temperature to prevent abdominal cramping.

   E. **CORRECT:** The nurse should inspect the tube insertion site for manifestations of infection, skin or mucosal breakdown, and leakage each time the client receives a bolus feeding.

   (N) *NCLEX® Connection: Basic Care and Comfort, Nutrition and Oral Hydration*

5. A. The feeding bag should be filled with only enough formula for 4 hr to prevent bacterial contamination.

   B. **CORRECT:** Feeding equipment, such as the bag holding the formula and the tubing, should be discarded every 24 hr to prevent bacterial contamination.

   C. The unused portion of formula should be refrigerated up to 24 hr to prevent bacterial contamination.

   D. **CORRECT:** The unused portion of the formula should be labeled with the time and date the formula was opened and the client's name and room number.

   E. The nurse should elevate the head of the client's bed for 30 to 60 min following administration to prevent aspiration.

   (N) *NCLEX® Connection: Basic Care and Comfort, Nutrition and Oral Hydration*

PRACTICE Answer

Using the ATI Active Learning Template: Basic Concept

RELATED CONTENT

Gastrointestinal disturbance
- Increase the amount of free fluid if constipated.
- Consider a change to formula with enriched fiber if constipated.
- Decrease the flow rate if cramping occurs.
- Give the formula at room temperature.

Feeding tube obstruction
- Flush the tubing with 15 to 30 mL of warm water every 4 hr.
- Flush before and after feedings and medication.
- Use a piston syringe with 50 mL of warm water to unclog the tubing.
- Only use a carbonated beverage if warm water does not open the tubing.

Food poisoning
- Wash hands before handling the formula or equipment.
- Clean tops of formula containers.
- Cover, label, and refrigerate formula up to 24 hr.
- Replace the feeding bag and administration tubing every 24 hr.

(N) *NCLEX® Connection: Reduction of Risk Potential, Potential for Complications of Diagnostic Tests/Treatments/Procedures*

CHAPTER 10 *Total Parenteral Nutrition*

Parenteral nutrition (PN) is used when a client's gastrointestinal tract is not functioning, or when a client cannot physically or psychologically consume sufficient nutrients orally or enterally. Based upon the client's nutritional needs and anticipated duration of therapy, PN can be given as either total parenteral nutrition (TPN) or peripheral parenteral nutrition (PPN).

TPN provides a nutritionally complete solution. It can be used when caloric needs are very high, when the anticipated duration of therapy is greater than 7 days, or when the solution to be administered is hypertonic (composed of greater than 10% dextrose). It can only be administered in a central vein.

PPN can provide a nutritionally complete solution. However, it is administered into a peripheral vein, resulting in a limited nutritional value. It is indicated for clients who require short-term nutritional support with fewer calories per day. The solution must be isotonic and contain no more than 10% dextrose and 5% amino acids.

COMPONENTS OF PARENTERAL NUTRITION SOLUTIONS

PN includes amino acids, dextrose, electrolytes, vitamins, and trace elements in sterile water.

Carbohydrate or dextrose solutions are available in concentrations of 5% for PPN and up to 70% for TPN.
- A higher concentration of dextrose is often prescribed for a client on fluid restrictions.
- A lower-dextrose concentration may be used to help control hyperglycemia.

Electrolytes, vitamins, and trace elements are essential for normal body functions. The amounts added are dependent upon the client's blood chemistry values and physical findings which are used to determine the quantity of electrolytes. Additional vitamin K may be added to the PN solution.

Lipids (fats) are available in concentrations of 10%, 20%, and 30%. Lipids are a significant source of calories and are used to correct or prevent essential fatty acid deficiency. It is formulated from a combination of soybean oil and/or safflower oil, and egg phospholipids.
- Lipid emulsions can be added to the PN solution, administered piggyback, or given intermittently.
- IV lipids are contraindicated for clients who have hyperlipidemia, severe hepatic disease, or an allergy to soybean oil, eggs, or safflower oil.
- Lipid emulsion provides the needed calories when dextrose concentration must be reduced due to fluid restrictions or persistent hyperglycemia.
- Lipid emulsion provides the calories without increasing the osmolality of the PN solution.

Protein is provided as a mixture of essential and nonessential amino acids and is available in concentrations of 3.5% to 15%. The client's estimated requirements and liver and kidney function determine the amount of protein provided.

Two medications, **insulin and heparin**, may be added to the PN solution by pharmacy services. Insulin can be added to reduce the potential for hyperglycemia, and heparin can be added to prevent fibrin buildup on the catheter tip. Administering any IV medication through a PN IV line or port is contraindicated.

INDICATIONS

DIAGNOSES

- TPN is commonly used in clients who need intense nutritional support for an extended period of time, including clients undergoing treatment for cancer, bowel disorders, those who are critically ill, and those suffering from trauma or extensive burns, as these conditions are associated with high caloric requirements.
- PPN may be used when the client is unable to consume enough calories to meet metabolic needs or when nutritional support is needed for a short time period (7 to 10 days).

DESIRED THERAPEUTIC OUTCOMES

- Improved nutritional status
- Weight maintenance or gain
- Positive nitrogen balance

EVIDENCE SUPPORTING EFFECTIVENESS

- Daily weight: Maintenance of baseline or gain of up to 1 kg/day.
- Increases in albumin level (expected reference range of 3.5 to 5.0 g/dL) and in prealbumin level (expected reference range of 15 to 36 mg/dL).

CONSIDERATIONS

PREPARATION OF THE CLIENT

- Prior to initiating PN, review the client's weight, BMI, nutritional status, diagnosis, and current laboratory data. This can include CBC, serum chemistry profile, PT/aPTT, iron, total iron-binding capacity, lipid profile, liver function tests, electrolyte panel, BUN, prealbumin and albumin level, creatinine, blood glucose, and platelet count.
- Assess the client's educational needs.
- Use an electronic infusion device to prevent the accidental overload of a solution.
- A micron filter on the IV tubing is required when administering PN solution. This filter is not added to the IV tubing when administering a lipid emulsion. Follow facility guidelines when administering all PN solutions.
- Evaluate the client for the presence of allergies to soybeans, safflower, or eggs if lipids are prescribed.

ONGOING CARE

Nursing care is focused on preventing complications through consistent monitoring. Specific monitoring guidelines vary among health care facilities.

- Ongoing assessment parameters include I&O, daily weights, vital signs, pertinent laboratory values (e.g., serum electrolytes, blood glucose), and ongoing evaluation of the client's underlying condition. This data is used to determine the client's response to therapy and the formulation of the solution to prevent nutrient deficiencies or toxicities.
- Monitor serum and urine glucose as prescribed and per facility guidelines. Sliding scale insulin may be prescribed to intervene for hyperglycemia, or regular insulin can be added to the PN solution.
- Monitor flow rate carefully.
  - Failure to provide optimal nutritional intake is the result of solutions administered too slowly.
  - Hyperosmolar diuresis can result from an infusion that is too rapid, and can lead to dehydration, hypovolemic shock, seizures, coma, and death.
  - To avoid hypoglycemia, an IV of dextrose 10% to 20% in water is administered if the PN solution is unavailable.
  - Do not attempt to increase the rate of the PN solution to "catch up." Hyperglycemia, hyperosmolar diuresis, and fluid overload can occur if the PN solution is increased when available.
- Monitor for "cracking" of TPN solution. This occurs if the calcium or phosphorous content is high or if poor-salt albumin is added. A "cracked" TPN solution has an oily appearance or a layer of fat on top of the solution and should not be used. Qs
- Verify the prescription of the PN solution with a second nurse prior to administration.
- If the PN solution is prepared and stored in the refrigerator, allow it to come to room temperature for 1 hr prior to administering it.

- Maintain strict aseptic techniques to reduce the risk of infection. The high dextrose content of PN contributes to bacterial growth.
- Use sterile technique when changing central line dressing and tubing. The bag and tubing should be changed every 24 hr or per facility protocol.

NURSING ACTIONS

- PN should be discontinued as soon as possible to avoid potential complications, but not until the client's enteral or oral intake can provide 60% or more of estimated caloric requirements.

  ! Discontinuation should be done gradually to avoid rebound hypoglycemia.

- Education for clients and family regarding TPN at home begins with a psychosocial assessment to determine coping and readiness, and then should include aseptic preparation and administration techniques, blood glucose monitoring, and criteria to evaluate for the presence of infection and complications.

COMPLICATIONS

Infection and sepsis are evidenced by a fever or elevated WBC count. Infection can result from contamination of the catheter during insertion, contaminated solution, or a long-term indwelling catheter.

Metabolic complications include hyperglycemia, hypoglycemia, hyperkalemia, hypophosphatemia, hypocalcemia, dehydration (related to hyperosmolar diuresis resulting from hyperglycemia), and fluid overload (as evidenced by weight gain greater than 1 kg/day and edema).

Mechanical complications include catheter misplacement resulting in pneumothorax or hemothorax (evidenced by shortness of breath, diminished or absent breath sounds), arterial puncture, catheter embolus, air embolus, thrombosis, obstruction, and bolus infusion due to incorrectly set or malfunctioning electronic pumps.

NURSING ACTIONS

- Monitor for manifestations of fever, chills, increased WBCs, and redness around the catheter insertion site.
- Use strict aseptic technique when setting up the IV tubing and accessing or deaccessing the port.
  - Use sterile technique when changing central line dressing and tubing.
  - Change the PN bag and tubing set every 24 hr or per facility protocol.
- Monitor blood glucose per prescription or facility policy.
- Administer sliding scale insulin or plan for insulin to be added to the TPN solution to treat hyperglycemia.
- Plan to administer additional dextrose to treat hypoglycemia.
- Monitor daily weights, I&O, and oral intake of nutrients.
- Notify the provider of weight gain greater than 1 kg/day.
- Anticipate a decrease in the concentration of the solution, rate of administration, or volume of lipid emulsion to treat weight gain.

Application Exercises

1. A nurse is planning care for a client who has a new prescription for peripheral parenteral nutrition (PPN). Which of the following actions should the nurse include in the plan of care? (Select all that apply.)

   A. Examine trends in weight loss.

   B. Review prealbumin finding.

   C. Administer an IV solution of 20% dextrose.

   D. Add a micron filter to IV tubing.

   E. Use an IV infusion pump.

2. A charge nurse is providing information about fat emulsion added to total parenteral nutrition (TPN) to a group of nurses. Which of the following statements by the charge nurse are appropriate? (Select all that apply.)

   A. "Concentration of lipid emulsion can be up to 30%."

   B. "Adding lipid emulsion gives the solution a milky appearance."

   C. "Check for allergies to soybean oil."

   D. "Lipid emulsion prevents essential fatty acid deficiency."

   E. "Lipids provide calories by increasing the osmolality of the PN solution."

3. A charge nurse is teaching a group of nurses about medication compatibility with TPN. Which of the following statements should the charge nurse make?

   A. "Use the Y-port on the TPN IV tubing to administer antibiotics."

   B. "Regular insulin may be added to the TPN solution."

   C. "Administer heparin through a port on the TPN tubing."

   D. "Administer vitamin K IV bolus via a Y-port on the TPN tubing."

4. A nurse is preparing to administer lipid emulsion and notes a layer of fat floating in the IV solution bag. Which of the following actions should the nurse take?

   A. Shake the bag to mix the fat.

   B. Turn the bag upside down one time.

   C. Return the bag to the pharmacy.

   D. Administer the bag of solution.

5. A nurse is caring for a client who is receiving TPN through a central line, but the next bag of solution is not available for administration at this time. Which of the following is an appropriate action by the nurse?

   A. Administer 20% dextrose in water IV until the next bag is available.

   B. Slow the infusion rate of the current bag until the solution is available.

   C. Monitor for hyperglycemia.

   D. Monitor for hyperosmolar diuresis.

PRACTICE Active Learning Scenario

A nurse is teaching a client about complications that can occur when receiving total parenteral nutrition (TPN). What should the nurse include in the teaching? Use the ATI Active Learning Template: Basic Concept to complete this item to include the following.

RELATED CONTENT: Identify three complications of TPN. Describe two nursing actions related to each complication.

Application Exercises Key

1. A. **CORRECT:** Examining trends in weight loss will help to evaluate the outcome of PPN.

   B. **CORRECT:** Reviewing the prealbumin finding will determine nutritional deficiency over a short period of time.

   C. An IV solution of 20% dextrose is administered only as TPN using a central vein.

   D. **CORRECT:** A micron filter is always used when infusing PN solution.

   E. **CORRECT:** An IV infusion pump is always used to regulate the flow and provide accurate delivery of the PN solution.

   Ⓝ *NCLEX® Connection: Pharmacological and Parenteral Therapies, Total Parenteral Nutrition (TPN)*

2. A. **CORRECT:** Lipid emulsion is available in 10%, 20%, and 30% concentrations depending upon the client's carbohydrate and caloric needs.

   B. **CORRECT:** The lipid emulsion is formulated from safflower and/or soybean oils and egg phospholipid, making the solution appear milky.

   C. **CORRECT:** Lipid emulsion is formulated from safflower and/or soybean oil and egg phospholipid. The nurse should check for allergies to these ingredients.

   D. **CORRECT:** Lipid emulsion is used for additional calories as concentrated energy and to prevent essential fatty acid deficiency.

   E. Lipids provide the calories needed without increasing osmolality of the PN solution.

   Ⓝ *NCLEX® Connection: Pharmacological and Parenteral Therapies, Total Parenteral Nutrition (TPN)*

3. A. Administering any IV medication through a Y-port on the TPN line is contraindicated.

   B. **CORRECT:** Regular insulin may be added to the TPN solution to decrease hyperglycemia.

   C. Heparin may be added to the TPN solution to decrease clot formation in the cannula, but it is not injected directly into a port on the TPN tubing.

   D. Vitamin K can be added to the TPN solution, but it should not be administered IV bolus through the TPN IV line.

   Ⓝ *NCLEX® Connection: Pharmacological and Parenteral Therapies, Total Parenteral Nutrition (TPN)*

4. A. Shaking the bag is not an appropriate action because "cracking" of the solution has occurred and it should not be administered.

   B. Turning the solution upside down does not resolve the problem because "cracking" of the TPN has occurred and it should not be administered.

   C. **CORRECT:** Returning the solution to the pharmacy is an appropriate action by the nurse because "cracking" of the solution has occurred and it should not be administered.

   D. Administering the solution is not an appropriate nursing action because "cracking" of the solution has occurred. Infusion of a cracked solution can lead to fat or particulate embolisms.

   Ⓝ *NCLEX® Connection: Pharmacological and Parenteral Therapies, Nutrition and Oral Hydration*

5. A. **CORRECT:** Administering 20% dextrose in water IV until the TPN solution is available will prevent hypoglycemia.

   B. Decreasing the rate of the TPN solution is not an appropriate action because the decreased rate can cause hypoglycemia.

   C. The client should be monitored for hypoglycemia when the TPN solution is not infusing and adequate glucose is not provided.

   D. The nurse should monitor the client for hyperosmolar diuresis when the TPN solution has infused too fast.

   Ⓝ *NCLEX® Connection: Pharmacological and Parenteral Therapies, Total Parenteral Nutrition (TPN)*

PRACTICE Answer

Using the ATI Active Learning Template: Basic Concept

RELATED CONTENT

Infection and sepsis
- Monitor for manifestations of fever, chills, increased WBCs, and redness around catheter insertion site.
- Use aseptic technique when setting up the IV tubing and accessing or deaccessing the port.
- Use sterile technique when changing central line dressing and tubing.
- Change the PN bag and tubing set every 24 hr or per facility protocol.

Hyperglycemia
- Administer sliding scale insulin or plan for insulin to be added to the TPN solution.
- Monitor blood glucose.

Hypoglycemia
- Inform the provider and plan to give additional dextrose.
- Monitor frequent blood glucose.

Weight gain greater than 1 kg/day
- Inform the provider and anticipate a decrease in the concentration, rate of administration or volume of lipid emulsion.
- Monitor the client's intake of oral nutrients.

Ⓝ *NCLEX® Connection: Pharmacological and Parenteral Therapies, Nutrition and Oral Hydration*

When reviewing the following chapters, keep in mind the relevant topics and tasks of the NCLEX outline, in particular:

Client Needs: Health Promotion and Maintenance

HEALTH PROMOTION/DISEASE PREVENTION:
Identify risk factors for disease/illness.

HEALTH SCREENING: Perform targeted screening assessments.

HIGH-RISK BEHAVIORS: Assist the client to identify behaviors/risks that may impact health.

Client Needs: Basic Care and Comfort

NUTRITION AND ORAL HYDRATION
Provide nutritional supplements as needed.

Evaluate the impact of disease/illness on the nutritional status of a client.

Client Needs: Physiological Adaptation

ALTERATIONS IN BODY SYSTEMS: Implement interventions to address side/adverse effects of radiation therapy.

ILLNESS MANAGEMENT: Educate the client about managing illness.

FLUID AND ELECTROLYTE IMBALANCES: Manage the care of the client with a fluid and electrolyte imbalance.

Many individuals have difficulty consuming a nutritional or prescribed diet due to factors that create a barrier. Medical, psychological, and social factors can all create nutritional barriers. Up to 40% of clients in acute care facilities are malnourished either upon admission or throughout a period of their hospital stay.

It is important for nurses to recognize these factors as nutritional education will be ineffective if a client lacks the necessary resources to follow through on recommendations.

NUTRITIONAL BARRIERS AND NURSING INTERVENTIONS

Poor dentition

Poor dentition (dental caries, poorly fitting dentures) is a potential problem for clients across the lifespan.
- Children who do not have access to dental care or tools (toothbrush, toothpaste) can have caries that impair the ability to chew.
- Adults who have lost teeth or have teeth that need removal or repair have an impaired ability to chew.
- After an adult has teeth removed, it can be difficult to adjust to dentures.

NURSING CARE
- School screenings can help identify children who need dental attention, and can facilitate the referral process.
- Provide children with information about healthy snacks that are low in sugar.
- Advise children and adults to limit consumption of processed carbohydrates, which can stick to teeth and increase the risk for dental caries.
- Encourage children and adults to use a fluoridated tooth paste and have fluoride applied to their teeth. Q𝐄𝐁𝐏
- Adults who are admitted to acute or long-term care facilities should have a dental inspection done by a nurse to identify issues that can affect the ability to properly eat.
- If a barrier is found to exist, consult a dietitian so the proper diet is prescribed and nutritional supplements are added as necessary.

Low socioeconomic status and lack of access

The lack of money to purchase healthy foods or foods required for a specific diet can be a barrier to maintaining a proper diet.
- Nutritious foods (fresh fruit, vegetables) tend to be more expensive than canned and boxed foods.
- Canned, boxed, and processed foods such as lunch meats and frozen meals are usually high in calories and salt, and often contain a higher fat, sodium, and simple carbohydrate content. These are poor choices for clients on calorie- or sodium-restricted diets.
- The lack of money to purchase necessary food can lead to malnutrition or obesity if canned and boxed foods are selected.
- The lack of transportation to grocery stores is a barrier if the client does not have a car or is not licensed to drive.

NURSING CARE
- Refer the client to a dietitian who can discuss food options and substitutions that are appropriate.
- Frozen fruits and vegetables can be an affordable option, and are maintained longer in the freezer.
- Educate clients on how to read food labels to be aware of nutritional, caloric, and sodium values of the food they are consuming.
- Contact social services regarding the availability of food or meal delivery to the client's home. Investigate the availability of a nutrition program that provides a noon meal for older adults within a community. Q𝐓𝐂

Cognitive disorders

Cognitive disorders (dementia, Alzheimer's disease [AD]) can have a significant impact on nutritional status.
- Clients who have dementia or AD can experience impairments in memory and judgment, making shopping, food selection, and food preparation difficult.
- As dementia and AD progress, clients might refuse to eat or choose a small selection of food that might not provide adequate nutrition.

NURSING CARE
- If the client lives independently, encourage shopping with a friend or family member, and to follow a shopping list.
- Monitor for vitamin and mineral deficits, and evaluate the need for nutritional supplements.
- Contact social services regarding the availability of food or meal delivery to the client's home.
- If the client lives in a care facility, provide a menu with minimal but nutritious options.
- Serve meals at the same time and in the same location surrounded by the same people. Keep environmental distractions to a minimum.
- Provide snacks in between meals if meal time intake is inadequate.
- Cut food into small pieces if the client does has difficulty chewing food. Remind the client to chew and then swallow. Lightly stroking the chin and throat can help promote swallowing. Q𝐒

Altered sensory perception

Clients who have an alteration in vision, smell, or taste can find it difficult to feed themselves or can find food unpalatable.

- Clients who have decreased vision might need assistance shopping for food on a regular basis, and with food preparation.
- Clients in a health care or long-term care facility might need help with tray setup and location of food on the tray.
- Clients who have an altered sense of smell have an altered sense of taste.
- Clients who smoke might have a diminished sense of smell.
- Clients on chemotherapy and other types of medications can have an unusual metallic taste in their mouth, masking the real taste of food.
- Clients receiving radiation to the head and neck can experience altered or loss of taste (mouth blindness).

NURSING CARE

- Encourage the client who has decreased vision to shop with a friend or family member, or have groceries delivered to the house. Q PCC
- Contact social services regarding availability of food or meal delivery to the client's home.
- Recommend to the client who has a food aversion to eat foods that are served cool, as they are typically less aromatic and are less likely to precipitate nausea.
- Suggest consuming foods that are spicy or tangy to compensate for the decreased sense of taste.
- Recommend sucking on hard candies, mints, or chewing gum to counteract an unusual taste in the mouth.
- Instruct the client to avoid ingestion of empty calories. If an increase in calories and fluid is desired, milkshakes, juice, and supplements are good options.

Impairment in swallowing

Clients who have neurological disorders (Parkinson's disease, cerebral palsy, stroke) or had a surgical procedure done on their mouth, throat, epiglottis, or larynx can have difficulty managing food and swallowing without choking.

- Clients who have a neurological disorder affecting the muscles in the mouth and throat are at risk for aspiration due to delayed swallowing and/or inadequate mastication.
- Clients who have a history of oral cancer might have had part of their lip, tongue, and/or soft palate removed. This significantly affects the ability to masticate and coordinate the development of a bolus of food prior to swallowing.
- Clients who have had their epiglottis completely or partially removed, or part of their larynx removed, have an anatomical structure removed that previously prevented food from entering the trachea. Unless precautions are taken, the client will easily aspirate food and fluids.

NURSING CARE

- Continually monitor clients who are at risk for aspiration during meals, and have suction equipment immediately available. Q S
- Consult a dietitian regarding an appropriate diet for the client (thick liquids, pureed, mechanical soft).
- Thicken thin fluids with a commercial thickener to the prescribed consistency of a nectar, honey, or pudding.
- Allow adequate time for assisting the client who has dysphagia to eat.
- Teach clients who aspirate easily due to surgical alteration of their throat or upper tracheal structures to tuck their chins when swallowing. Arching the tongue in the back of the throat can help close off the trachea.

Mechanical fixation of the jaw

Disorders of the jaw requiring surgery include facial trauma and reconstruction.

- After fractured bones are realigned, the client's upper and lower jaw can be wired together.
- The jaw can be immobilized for several weeks.
- The client is generally placed on a liquid diet during this period.

NURSING CARE

- Encourage the intake of fluids.
- Help the client determine where to insert a straw through the space between the jaws.
- Work with the dietitian to develop a liquid meal plan that includes the necessary nutrients. Q TC

Lack of knowledge and misinformation about nutrition

Clients who do not have a good understanding about nutritional needs can be subject to overnutrition, undernutrition, and the ingestion of an inadequate intake of essential nutrients.

- Clients might not have basic knowledge about nutrition.
- Information about nutrition can be confusing or misleading.
- Clients can be drawn to fad diets (which are generally unhealthy) because quick results are promised.
- Clients can be misled by false advertising.

NURSING CARE

- Encourage clients to use dietary guidelines available from government and health associations (MyPlate [www.choosemyplate.gov], the American Heart Association). Q EBP
- Assist clients in locating community resources that provide education on nutrition.
- Assess dietary intake.
- Instruct clients on how to read nutrition fact labels.
- Encourage the client to keep a journal of dietary intake.
- Provide clients with information on foods that are healthy and portion sizes.
- Warn clients that advertisements can be fraudulent.

Medical conditions

- Clients who have medical conditions such as cancer, COPD, burns, severe trauma, or HIV/AIDS are at increased risk for malnutrition due to anorexia, nausea, or stomatitis related to treatments, increased metabolic demands, or the ability to consume a diet.
- Clients who are undergoing diagnostic testing that require NPO status are potentially at risk.
- Clients who have comorbidities resulting in polypharmacy are at risk for malnutrition and medication nutrient interactions.

NURSING CARE

- Monitor diet prescriptions and laboratory results, particularly for clients who are receiving clear or full liquid diets for more than 24 hr. Refer the client to a dietitian for a complete evaluation of nutritional status. Q_{TC}
- Monitor clients who have comorbidities for interactions between medications and nutrition. Refer the client to a pharmacist for a thorough evaluation of medication interactions and the impact upon nutritional intake.

- Offer several small meals or snacks through the day instead of three large meals.
- Provide oral care prior to and following meals.
- Discourage the use of alcohol-based mouthwashes for clients who have stomatitis.
- Provide liquid supplements between meals to increase nutrient intake.

PRACTICE Active Learning Scenario

A nurse is providing dietary teaching for a client who requests assistance for weight loss. The client states, "I've tried several fad diets but they don't work for me." Use the ATI Active Learning Template: Basic Concept to complete this item to include the following sections.

UNDERLYING PRINCIPLES: Identify the client's barrier to nutrition.

NURSING INTERVENTIONS: Identify at least four interventions to address this client's barrier to nutrition and to promote healthy weight loss.

Application Exercises

1. A nurse is caring for several clients in an extended care facility. Which of the following clients is the highest priority to observe during meals?
   - A. A client who has decreased vision
   - B. A client who has Parkinson's disease
   - C. A client who has poor dentition
   - D. A client who has anorexia

2. A nurse is planning care for an older adult client who is receiving treatment for malnutrition. The client is scheduled for discharge to his home where he lives alone. Which of the following actions should the nurse include in the plan of care? (Select all that apply.)
   - A. Consult social services to arrange home meal delivery.
   - B. Encourage the client to purchase nonperishable boxed meals.
   - C. Advise the client to purchase frozen fruits and vegetables.
   - D. Recommend drinking a supplement between meals.
   - E. Educate the client on how to read nutrition labels.

3. A nurse is providing teaching for a client who has a new diagnosis of hypertension and a prescription for a low-sodium diet. Which of the following client statements indicate an understanding of the teaching? (Select all that apply.)
   - A. "I should select organic canned vegetables."
   - B. "I need to read food labels when grocery shopping."
   - C. "I will stop eating frozen dinners for lunch at work."
   - D. "I know that deli meats are usually high in sodium."
   - E. "I can refer to the American Heart Association's website for dietary guidelines."

4. A nurse is caring for a client who is transitioning to an oral diet following a partial laryngectomy. Which of the following actions should the nurse take to reduce the client's risk for aspiration?
   - A. Request to have the client's oral medications provided in liquid form.
   - B. Instruct the client to follow each bite of food with a drink of water.
   - C. Encourage the client to tuck the chin when swallowing.
   - D. Consult the dietitian about providing the client with a thin liquid diet.

5. A nurse is planning care for a client who has mechanical fixation of the jaw following a motorcycle crash. Which of the following actions should the nurse include in the plan of care? (Select all that apply.)
   - A. Thicken liquids to honey consistency.
   - B. Educate the client about the use of a nasogastric tube.
   - C. Assist the client to use a straw to drink liquids.
   - D. Ensure that the client receives ground meats.
   - E. Encourage intake of fluids between meals.

Application Exercises Key

1. A. Observation of a client who has decreased vision is necessary to evaluate the client's need for assistance. However, this client is not the highest priority to observe during meals.

   B. **CORRECT:** A client who has Parkinson's disease is at risk for aspiration. Due to this safety risk, this client is the highest priority to observe during meals.

   C. Observation of a client who has poor dentition is necessary to evaluate the client's need for assistance or a modified diet. However, this client is not the highest priority to observe during meals.

   D. Observation of a client who has anorexia is necessary to evaluate the client's intake. However, this client is not the highest priority to observe during meals.

   (N) *NCLEX® Connection: Safety and Infection Control, Accident/Error/Injury Prevention*

2. A. **CORRECT:** The nurse should consult social services to arrange home meal delivery to promote adequate nutrition.

   B. Boxed foods are usually high in calories and salt and are therefore not recommended to promote adequate nutrition.

   C. **CORRECT:** The nurse should advise the client to purchase frozen fruits and vegetables to promote adequate nutrition.

   D. **CORRECT:** The nurse should recommend a supplement between meals to promote adequate nutrition.

   E. **CORRECT:** The nurse should educate the client on how to read food labels to promote adequate nutrition.

   (N) *NCLEX® Connection: Physiological Adaptation, Illness Management*

3. A. Canned foods, even if organic, are usually high in sodium and are therefore a poor choice for a client on a sodium-restricted diet.

   B. **CORRECT:** Reading food labels provides the client with information about the food's sodium content.

   C. Frozen dinners are usually high in sodium and are therefore a poor choice for a client on a sodium-restricted diet.

   D. **CORRECT:** Deli meats are usually high in sodium and are therefore a poor choice for a client on a sodium-restricted diet.

   E. **CORRECT:** The American Heart Association is a recommended health association for continued client education on dietary guidelines related to cardiac disorders such as hypertension.

   (N) *NCLEX® Connection: Physiological Adaptation, Illness Management*

4. A. Providing medications in liquid form does not decrease the risk for aspiration.

   B. Drinking thin liquids, such as water, increases the risk for aspiration.

   C. **CORRECT:** Tucking the chin when swallowing helps to close off the trachea and reduces the risk for aspiration.

   D. Thick, rather than thin, liquids help reduce the risk for aspiration.

   (N) *NCLEX® Connection: Reduction of Risk Potential, Potential for Complications of Diagnostic Tests/Treatments/Procedures*

5. A. Mechanical fixation of the jaw does not cause dysphagia. It is not necessary to thicken the client's liquids.

   B. Mechanical fixation of the jaw does not indicate the need for a nasogastric tube.

   C. **CORRECT:** The nurse should recommend the use of a straw to drink liquids. The nurse should help the client determine where to insert the straw through the space between the jaws.

   D. Mechanical fixation of the jaw indicates the need for a liquid diet rather than ground meats.

   E. **CORRECT:** The client who has a mechanical fixation of the jaw will have the jaws wired shut and is only able to consume liquids. The nurse should encourage supplemental and nutrient-rich liquids to maintain adequate hydration and nutrition.

   (N) *NCLEX® Connection: Basic Care and Comfort, Nutrition and Oral Hydration*

PRACTICE Answer

Using the ATI Active Learning Template: Basic Concept

UNDERLYING PRINCIPLES: The client's barrier to nutrition is lack of knowledge and misinformation about nutrition. This barrier must be acknowledged to promote adequate nutrition.

NURSING INTERVENTIONS
- Encourage the client to use dietary guidelines such as MyPlate.
- Assist the client in locating community resources that provide education and nutrition to support healthy nutrition and weight loss.
- Advise the clients that fad diets are generally unhealthy and often include false advertising.
- Perform an assessment of dietary intake.
- Encourage the client to keep a journal of dietary intake.
- Provide the client with information on healthy foods and portion sizes.

(N) *NCLEX® Connection: Health Promotion and Maintenance, Health Promotion/Disease Prevention*

UNIT 3   ALTERATIONS IN NUTRITION

CHAPTER 12 *Cardiovascular and Hematologic Disorders*

Nurses must have an awareness of nutritional needs for clients who have cardiovascular and hematologic disorders. It is important to explore dietary needs with the client and recommend modifications related to the disease process. Understanding the role of primary and secondary prevention is essential to successful treatment.

Cardiovascular diseases are the leading cause of death in the United States. Coronary heart disease (CHD) is the single leading cause of death.

ASSESSMENT/DATA COLLECTION

Coronary heart disease

Hypercholesterolemia is a major risk factor for developing CHD. CHD is caused by atherosclerosis, a process of damage and cholesterol deposits on the blood vessels of the heart.
- High-density lipoprotein (HDL) cholesterol is "good" cholesterol because it removes cholesterol from the serum and takes it to the liver. Levels greater than or equal to 60 mg/dL provide some protection against heart disease.
- Low-density lipoprotein (LDL) cholesterol is "bad" cholesterol because it transports cholesterol out of the liver and into the circulatory system, where it can form plaques on the coronary artery walls. The optimal range for LDL is less than 130 mg/dL.
- Optimal total cholesterol level is less than 200 mg/dL. ⓠEBP

RISK FACTORS
- **NONMODIFIABLE**: increasing age, male gender, family history of early CHD
- **MODIFIABLE**: high LDL cholesterol, low HDL cholesterol, consuming a diet high in saturated fat, hypertension, diabetes mellitus, obesity, sedentary lifestyle, nicotine use disorder

Metabolic syndrome

The presence of three of the five following risk factors.
- Abdominal obesity
  - **MEN**: greater than or equal to 40-inch waist (greater than 35 inches for Asian men)
  - **WOMEN**: greater than or equal to 35-inch waist (greater than 31 inches for Asian women)
- Triglycerides greater than or equal to 150 mg/dL
- Low HDL
  - **MEN**: less than or equal to 40 mg/dL
  - **WOMEN**: less than or equal to 50 mg/dL
- Increased blood pressure
  - Systolic greater than or equal to 130 mm/Hg
  - Diastolic greater than or equal to 85 mm/Hg
- Fasting blood glucose greater than or equal to 100 mg/dL

ANEMIAS

Iron deficiency anemia

RISK FACTORS
- Blood loss, deficient iron intake from diet, alcohol use disorder, malabsorption syndromes, gastrectomy
- Metabolic increase caused by pregnancy, adolescence, infection

MANIFESTATIONS
- Fatigue
- Lethargy
- Pallor of nail beds
- Intolerance to cold
- Headache
- Tachycardia

! Children who have low iron intake can experience short attention spans and display poor intellectual performance before anemia begins.

Vitamin B₁₂ deficiency anemia (macrocytic)

RISK FACTORS: Lack of meat or dairy consumption, small bowel resection, chronic diarrhea, diverticula, tapeworm, excess of intestinal bacteria

MANIFESTATIONS
- Pallor
- Jaundice
- Weakness
- Fatigue

GASTROINTESTINAL FINDINGS
- Glossitis (inflamed tongue)
- Anorexia
- Indigestion
- Weight loss
- Frequent diarrhea and/or constipation

NEUROLOGICAL FINDINGS
- Decreased concentration
- Paresthesia (numbness) of hands and feet
- Decreased proprioception (sense of body position)
- Poor muscle coordination
- Increasing irritability
- Delirium

Folic acid deficiency anemia

RISK FACTORS: Poor nutritional intake of foods containing folic acid (green leafy vegetables, citrus fruits, dried bean, nuts), malabsorption syndromes such as Crohn's disease, certain medications such as anticonvulsants and oral contraceptives

MANIFESTATIONS

- Fatigue
- Pallor
- Glossitis
- Irritability
- Diarrhea

Findings of folic acid deficiency anemia mimic those for vitamin B_{12} deficiency anemia except for the neurological manifestations.

NUTRITIONAL GUIDELINES AND NURSING INTERVENTIONS

Coronary heart disease

PREVENTATIVE NUTRITION

- Consuming a low-fat, low-cholesterol diet can reduce the risk of developing CHD. The Therapeutic Lifestyle Change (TLC) diet is designed to be a user-friendly eating guide to encourage dietary changes.
- Daily cholesterol intake should be less than 200 mg.
- Conservative use of red wine can reduce the risk of developing CHD.
- Increasing fiber and carbohydrate intake, avoiding saturated fat, and decreasing red meat consumption can decrease the risk for developing CHD.
- Increased intake of omega-3 fatty acids found in fish, flaxseed, soy beans, canola, and walnuts reduces the risk of coronary artery disease.
- Homocysteine is an amino acid. Elevated homocysteine levels can increase the risk of developing CHD. Deficiencies in folate and vitamins B_6 and B_{12} increase homocysteine levels.

THERAPEUTIC NUTRITION

- Secondary prevention efforts for CHD are focused on lifestyle changes that lower LDL. These include a diet low in cholesterol and saturated fats, a diet high in fiber, exercise and weight management, and cessation of nicotine use.
- Daily cholesterol intake should be less than 200 mg/day. Saturated fat should be limited to less than 7% of daily caloric intake.
- To lower cholesterol and saturated fats, instruct the client to do the following.
  - Trim visible fat from meats.
  - Limit red meats and choose lean meats (turkey, chicken).
  - Remove the skin from meats.
  - Broil, bake, grill, or steam foods. Avoid frying foods.
  - Use low-fat or nonfat milk, cheese, and yogurt.
  - Use spices in place of butter or salt to season foods.
  - Use liquid oils such as olive or canola in place of oils that contain saturated fat.

- Avoid trans fat, which increases LDL. Partially hydrogenated products contain trans fat.
  - Increase consumption of oily fish (tuna, salmon, herring).
  - Read labels.
- Encourage the client to consume a high-fiber diet.
  - Soluble fiber lowers LDL.
  - Oats, beans, fruits, vegetables, whole grains, barley, and flaxseed are good sources of fiber.
- Encourage the client to exercise.
  - Instruct the client regarding practical methods for increasing physical activity. (Encourage the client to take the stairs rather than the elevator.)
  - Provide the client with references for local exercise facilities.
- Instruct the client to stop all use of tobacco products.
- The recommended lifestyle changes represent a significant change for many clients. Qᴘᴄᴄ
  - Provide support to the client and family.
  - Encourage the client's family to participate in the changes to ease the transition for the client.
  - Explain why the diet is important.
  - Aid the client in developing a diet that is complementary to personal food preferences and lifestyle. A food diary can be helpful.
  - Instruct the client that occasional deviations from the diet are reasonable.

Hypertension

- Hypertension is a significant risk factor for developing CHD, myocardial infarction, and stroke.
- Hypertension is a sustained elevation in blood pressure greater than or equal to 140/90 mm Hg for clients under the age of 60, 150/90 mm Hg for those older than 60.

RISK FACTORS FOR PRIMARY HYPERTENSION: family history, hyperlipidemia, smoking, obesity, physical inactivity, high sodium intake, low potassium intake, excessive alcohol consumption, stress, and aging. African-American people have the highest incidence of hypertension. A woman's risk of hypertension increases after menopause.

THERAPEUTIC NUTRITION

- The Dietary Approaches to Stopping Hypertension (DASH) diet is a low-sodium, high-potassium, high-calcium diet that has proven to lower blood pressure (systolic and diastolic) and cholesterol.
  - Decrease sodium intake (initially a daily intake of less than 2,300 mg is recommended, and should gradually be decreased to 1,500 mg for maximum benefit).
  - Foods high in sodium include canned soups and sauces, potato chips, pretzels, smoked meats, seasonings, and processed foods.
  - Include low-fat dairy products to promote calcium intake.
  - Include fruits and vegetables rich in potassium (apricots, bananas, tomatoes, potatoes).
- Limit alcohol intake.
- Encourage the client to read labels and educate the client about appropriate food choices.
- Other lifestyle changes include exercising, weight loss, and smoking cessation.

Heart failure

Heart failure is characterized by the inability of the heart to maintain adequate blood flow throughout the circulatory system. It results in excess sodium and fluid retention, and edema.

RISK FACTORS: CHD, arrhythmias, previous MI, valve disorders, hypertension, obesity, diabetes, and metabolic syndrome

THERAPEUTIC NUTRITION
- Reduce sodium intake to 2,000 mg/day or less.
- Monitor fluid intake (and possibly restrict 2 L/day).
- Increase protein intake to 1.12 g/kg.
- Small, frequent meals that are soft, easy-to-chew foods.

Myocardial infarction

- A myocardial infarction (MI) occurs when there is an inadequate supply of oxygen to the myocardium. Frequently, an MI occurs because of atherosclerosis.
- After an MI, it is necessary to reduce the myocardial oxygen demands related to metabolic activity.
- Risk factors for MI are the same as for CHD.

THERAPEUTIC NUTRITION
- A liquid diet is best for the first 24 hr after the infarction.
- Caffeine should be avoided because it stimulates the heart and increases heart rate.
- Small, frequent meals are indicated.
- Counsel the client about recommendations for a heart-healthy diet.

Anemia

Anemia results from either a reduction in the number of red blood cells (RBCs) or in hemoglobin, the oxygen-carrying component of blood. Anemia can result from a decrease in RBC production, an increase in RBC destruction, or a loss of blood.
- The body requires iron, vitamin B_{12}, and folic acid to produce red blood cells.
- Iron deficiency anemia is the most common nutritional disorder in the world. It affects approximately 10% of the U.S. population, especially older infants, toddlers, adolescent girls, and pregnant women.
- From childhood until adolescence, iron intake tends to be marginal.
- Pernicious anemia is the most common form of vitamin B_{12} deficiency. It is caused by lack of intrinsic factor, a protein that helps the body absorb vitamin B_{12}.

SOURCES OF IRON
- Meat
- Fish
- Poultry
- Tofu
- Dried peas and beans
- Whole grains
- Dried fruit
- Iron-fortified foods
  - Infant formula (acceptable alternative or supplement to breastfeeding)
  - Infant cereal (usually the first food introduced to infants)
  - Ready-to-eat cereals

VITAMIN C: Facilitates the absorption of iron (promote consumption).

! Medicinal iron overdose is the leading cause of accidental poisoning in small children and can lead to acute iron toxicity. Qs

NATURAL SOURCES OF VITAMIN B_{12}
- Fish
- Meat
- Poultry
- Eggs
- Milk

People over the age of 50 are urged to consume most of their vitamin B_{12} requirement from supplements or fortified food.

Vegans need supplemental B_{12}.

FOLIC ACID SOURCES
- Green leafy vegetables
- Dried peas and beans
- Seeds
- Orange juice
- Cereals and breads fortified with folic acid

If the client is unable to obtain an adequate supply of folic acid, supplementation can be necessary.

1. A nurse is teaching a client about dietary recommendations to lower high blood pressure. Which of the following statements by the client indicates an understanding of the teaching ?

   A. "My daily sodium consumption should be 3,000 milligrams."

   B. "I should consume foods low in potassium."

   C. "My limit is three cigarettes a day."

   D. "I should consume low-fat dairy products."

2. A nurse is teaching a client about high-fiber foods that can assist in lowering LDL. Which of the following foods should the nurse include in the teaching? (Select all that apply.)

   A. Beans

   B. Cheese

   C. Whole grains

   D. Broccoli

   E. Yogurt

3. A community health nurse is assessing a client who reports numbness of the hands and feet for the past 2 weeks. This finding is associated with which of the following nutritional deficiencies?

   A. Folic acid

   B. Potassium

   C. Vitamin B_{12}

   D. Iron

4. A nurse is reviewing a client health record that includes a report of weight gain in the abdomen and laboratory findings of elevated blood glucose and elevated triglycerides. The nurse should identify that these findings are manifestations of which of the following conditions?

   A. Anemia

   B. Metabolic syndrome

   C. Heart failure

   D. Hypertension

5. A nurse is providing teaching to a client who has vitamin B_{12} deficiency. Which of the following foods should the nurse instruct the client to consume? (Select all that apply.)

   A. Meat

   B. Flaxseed

   C. Beans

   D. Eggs

   E. Milk

PRACTICE Active Learning Scenario

A nurse is providing teaching to a client who has hypertension. What should the nurse include in the teaching? Use the ATI Active Learning Template: System Disorder to complete this item to include the following sections.

ALTERATION IN HEALTH (DIAGNOSIS)

CLIENT EDUCATION: Describe the Dietary Approaches to Stopping Hypertension (DASH) diet and four nutrition teaching points to include..

Application Exercises Key

1. A. Daily sodium consumption should be 2,300 mg or less. This assists with lowering systolic and diastolic blood pressures as well as cholesterol.

    B. Foods high in potassium should be encouraged. This assists with lowering systolic and diastolic blood pressures as well as cholesterol.

    C. Smoking cessation should be encouraged. Smoking can increase blood pressure and should be avoided.

    D. **CORRECT:** Low-fat dairy products should be encouraged. They promote calcium intake and assist with lowering systolic and diastolic blood pressures as well as cholesterol.

    (N) *NCLEX® Connection: Basic Care and Comfort, Nutrition and Oral Hydration*

2. A. **CORRECT:** Beans are a food source high in fiber and should be included in the teaching.

    B. Cheese is a food source high in calcium and should not be included in the teaching.

    C. **CORRECT:** Whole grains are a food source high in fiber and should be included in the teaching.

    D. **CORRECT:** Broccoli is a food source high in fiber and should be included in the teaching.

    E. Yogurt is a food source high in calcium and should not be included in the teaching.

    (N) *NCLEX® Connection: Basic Care and Comfort, Nutrition and Oral Hydration*

3. A. Mental confusion, fatigue, fainting, and gastrointestinal distress are manifestations associated with folic acid deficiency.

    B. Irritability, decreased respirations, muscle weakness, and gastrointestinal distress are manifestations associated with hypokalemia.

    C. **CORRECT:** Numbness of the hands and feet are manifestations associated with vitamin B_{12} deficiency.

    D. Fatigue, lethargy, pallor of nail beds, and intolerance to cold are manifestations associated with iron deficiency anemia.

    (N) *NCLEX® Connection: Basic Care and Comfort, Nutrition and Oral Hydration*

4. A. Fatigue, lethargy, pallor of nail beds, and intolerance to cold are manifestations associated with anemia.

    B. **CORRECT:** Weight gain in the abdomen, elevated blood glucose, and elevated triglycerides are manifestations associated with metabolic syndrome.

    C. Shortness of breath, fluid retention, and fatigue are manifestations associated with heart failure.

    D. Headaches, tiredness, and dizziness are manifestations associated with hypertension.

    (N) *NCLEX® Connection: Basic Care and Comfort, Nutrition and Oral Hydration*

5. A. **CORRECT:** Meat is a food source that is high in vitamin B_{12}.

    B. Flaxseed is a good source of fiber.

    C. Beans are a good source of folic acid.

    D. **CORRECT:** Eggs are a food source that is high in vitamin B_{12}.

    E. **CORRECT:** Milk is a food source that is high in vitamin B_{12}.

    (N) *NCLEX® Connection: Basic Care and Comfort, Nutrition and Oral Hydration*

PRACTICE Answer

Using the ATI Active Learning Template: System Disorder

ALTERATION IN HEALTH (DIAGNOSIS): Hypertension is a sustained elevation in blood pressure greater than or equal to 140/90 mm Hg in clients less than age 60 and 150/90 mm Hg in those older than 60.

CLIENT EDUCATION
- The DASH diet is a low-sodium, high-potassium, high-calcium diet that has been proven to lower blood pressure and cholesterol.
- Lower sodium intake (daily intake of less than 2,300 mg) is recommended.
- Foods high in sodium include canned soups and sauces, potato chips, pretzels, smoked meats, seasonings, and processed foods.
- Include low-fat dairy products to promote calcium intake.
- Include fruits and vegetables rich in potassium (apricots, bananas, tomatoes, potatoes).
- Limit alcohol intake.

(N) *NCLEX® Connection: Physiological Adaptation, Illness Management*

UNIT 3   ALTERATIONS IN NUTRITION

CHAPTER 13 *Gastrointestinal Disorders*

Nurses must gain an awareness of nutritional needs for clients who have gastrointestinal (GI) disorders. It is important to explore dietary needs with the client and recommend modifications in relationship to the disease process. Understanding the role of primary and secondary prevention is essential to successful treatment.

Nutrition therapy for gastrointestinal disorders is generally aimed at minimizing or preventing manifestations. In some conditions, such as celiac disease, nutrition is the only treatment. For some GI disorders, nutrition therapy is the foundation of treatment.

ASSESSMENT/DATA COLLECTION

- Determine whether the client is experiencing any of the following.
  - Difficulty chewing or swallowing.
  - Nausea, vomiting, or diarrhea
  - Bloating, excessive flatus, occult blood, steatorrhea, abdominal pain or cramping, abdominal distention, pale, sticky bowel movements
  - Changes in weight, eating patterns, or bowel habits
- Determine whether the client uses the following.
  - Tobacco
  - Alcohol
  - Caffeine
  - Over-the-counter medications to treat GI conditions (many can have GI complications or be contradicted with GI conditions)
  - Nutritional supplements
  - Herbal supplements for GI conditions or other problems (some clients do not consider them to be medications, so they do not mention them to the provider)

NUTRITIONAL GUIDELINES AND NURSING INTERVENTIONS

General gastrointestinal considerations

- Monitor gastrointestinal parameters.
  - Weight and weight changes
  - Laboratory values
  - Elimination patterns
  - I&O
- Low-fiber diets avoid foods that are high in residue content (whole-grain breads and cereals, raw fruits and vegetables).
  - Diets low in fiber reduce the frequency and volume of fecal output and slow transit time of food through the digestive tract.
  - Low-fiber diets are used short-term for clients who have diarrhea or malabsorption syndromes.
- High-fiber diets focus on foods containing more than 5 g of fiber per serving. A diet high in fiber helps:
  - Increase stool bulk.
  - Stimulate peristalsis.
  - Prevent constipation.
  - Protect against colon cancer.

Nausea and vomiting

- Potential causes of nausea and vomiting include decreased gastric acid secretion; decreased gastrointestinal motility; allergy to food(s); bacterial or viral infection; increased intracranial pressure; liver, pancreatic, and gall bladder disorders; and adverse effects of some medications.
- The underlying cause of nausea and vomiting should be investigated. Assessing the appearance of the emesis will aid in diagnosis and treatment (e.g., coffee-ground emesis indicates the presence of blood; pale green indicates bile).
- Once manifestations subside, begin with clear liquids followed by full liquids, and advance the diet as tolerated.
- Easy-to-digest, low-fat carbohydrate foods (crackers, toast, oatmeal, pretzels, plain bread, bland fruit) are usually well-tolerated.

OTHER INTERVENTIONS
- Clients should avoid liquids with meals, as they promote a feeling of fullness.
- Promote good oral hygiene with tooth brushing, mouth swabs, mouthwash, and ice chips.
- Elevate the head of the bed.
- Discourage hot and spicy foods.
- Serve foods at room temperature or chilled.
- Avoid high-fat foods if they contribute to nausea because they are difficult to digest.

Anorexia

- Anorexia is defined as a lack of appetite. It is a common finding for numerous physical conditions and is an adverse effect of certain medications. It is not the same as anorexia nervosa.
- Anorexia can lead to decreased nutritional intake and subsequent protein and calorie deficits.

NURSING INTERVENTIONS
- Decrease stress at meal times.
- Collect data regarding adverse effects of medications.
- Administer medications to stimulate appetite.
- Assess and modify environment for unpleasant odors.
- Remove items that cause a decrease in appetite (soiled linens, garbage, emesis basins, bedpans, used tissues, clutter).
- Assess and manage anxiety and depression.
- Provide small, frequent meals and avoid high-fat foods to help maximize intake.
- Provide liquid supplements between meals to improve protein and calorie intake.
- Ensure that meals appear appealing. Serve larger meals early in the day.
- Assess for changes in bowel status (increased gastric emptying, constipation, diarrhea).
- Position to increase gastric motility.
- Provide mouth care before and after meals.

Constipation

- Clients who have constipation have difficult or infrequent passage of stools, which can be hard and dry.
- Causes include irregular bowel habits, psychogenic factors, inactivity, chronic laxative use, obstruction, medications, GI disorders such as irritable bowel syndrome (IBS), pregnancy, or secondary to genital/rectal trauma such as sexual abuse or childbirth, and inadequate consumption of fiber and fluid.
- Encourage exercise and a diet high in fiber (25 g/day for women and 38 g/day for men), and promote adequate fluid intake to help alleviate constipation.
- If caused by medication, a change in the medication might be necessary.

NURSING INTERVENTIONS
- Determine onset and duration of past and present elimination patterns, what is normal for the client, activity levels, occupation, dietary intake, and stress levels.
- Collect data about past medical and surgical history, medication use (OTC, herbal supplements, laxatives, enemas, and prescriptions), presence of rectal pressure or fullness, and abdominal pain.
- Encourage client to gradually increase daily intake of fiber.
- Advise the client that an increase in fiber intake is the preferred treatment for constipation. Chronic use of laxatives should be avoided.

Diarrhea

- Can cause significant losses of potassium, sodium, and fluid, as well as nutritional complications.
- Common causes of diarrhea include emotional and physical stress, gastrointestinal disorders, malabsorption disorders, infections, and certain medications.
- A high-fiber diet is often prescribed, unless fiber is causing the diarrhea.
- Nutrition therapy varies with the severity and duration of diarrhea. A liberal fluid intake to replace losses is needed.

Dysphagia

- Dysphagia is an alteration in the client's ability to swallow.
- Causes include obstruction, inflammation, and certain neurological disorders.
- Modifying the texture of foods and the consistency of liquids can enable the client to achieve proper nutrition.
- Dry mouth can contribute to dysphagia. Evaluate medications being taken to determine if this is a potential adverse effect.
- Clients who have dysphagia are at an increased risk of aspiration. Place the client in an upright or high-Fowler's position to facilitate swallowing. Qs
- Provide oral care prior to eating to enhance the client's sense of taste.
- Clients who have dysphagia should be referred to a speech therapist for evaluation.
- Dietary modifications are based on the specific swallowing limitations experienced by the client.
- Allow adequate time for eating, use adaptive eating devices, and encourage small bites and thorough chewing.
- Pills should be taken with at least 8 oz of fluid (can be thickened) to prevent medication from remaining in the esophagus.
- Avoid thin liquids and sticky foods.
- Nutritional supplements are beneficial if nutritional intake is deemed inadequate.

Dumping syndrome

Normally, the stomach controls the rate in which nutrients enter the small intestine. When a portion of the stomach is surgically removed, the contents of the stomach are rapidly emptied into the small intestine, causing dumping syndrome.
- Early manifestations typically occur 15 to 30 min after eating. Early manifestations include a sensation of fullness, abdominal cramping, nausea, diarrhea, and vasomotor manifestations (faintness, syncope, diaphoresis, tachycardia, hypotension, flushing).
- Late manifestations occur 1 to 3 hr after eating. Late manifestations include diaphoresis, weakness, tremors, anxiety, nausea, and hunger.
- Manifestations resolve after intestine is emptied. However, there is a rapid rise in blood glucose and increase in insulin levels immediately after the intestine empties. This leads to hypoglycemia.

NURSING INTERVENTIONS

- Recommend small, frequent meals.
- Recommend consuming protein and fat at each meal.
- Tell the client to avoid food that contains concentrated sugars and to restrict lactose intake.
- Suggest that the client consume liquids 1 hr before or after eating instead of during meals (dry diet).
- Instruct client to lie down for 20 to 30 min after meals to delay gastric emptying. If reflux is a problem, suggest a reclining position.
- Monitor clients receiving enteral tube feedings and report manifestations of dumping syndrome to the provider.
- Monitor the client for vitamin and mineral deficits, such as iron and vitamin B_{12}.

Gastroesophageal reflux disease

- Gastroesophageal reflux disease (GERD) occurs as the result of the abnormal reflux of gastric secretions up the esophagus. This leads to indigestion and heartburn.
- Factors that contribute to GERD include hiatal hernia, obesity, pregnancy, smoking, some medications, and genetics.
- Long-term GERD can cause serious complications, including adenocarcinoma of the esophagus and Barrett's esophagus.
- Manifestations include heartburn, retrosternal burning, painful swallowing, dyspepsia, regurgitation, coughing, hoarseness, and epigastric pain. Pain can be mistaken for a myocardial infarction.

NURSING INTERVENTIONS

- Instruct the client to avoid situations that lead to increased abdominal pressure, such as wearing tight-fitting clothing.
- Advise the client to avoid eating 2 hr or less before lying down.
- Advise the client to elevate the body on pillows instead of lying flat and to avoid large meals and bedtime snacks.
- Encourage weight loss for clients who are overweight.
- Suggest that the client avoid trigger foods (citrus fruits and juices, spicy foods, carbonated beverages).
- Instruct the client to avoid items that reduce lower esophageal sphincter pressure, including fatty foods, caffeine, chocolate, alcohol, cigarette smoke and all nicotine products, and peppermint and spearmint flavors.

Acute and chronic gastritis

- Gastritis is characterized by inflammation of the gastric mucosa. The gastric mucosa is congested with blood and fluid, becoming inflamed. There is a decrease in acid produced and an overabundance of mucus. Superficial ulcers occur, sometimes leading to hemorrhages.
- Acute gastritis occurs with excessive use of NSAIDs, bile reflux, ingestion of a strong acid or alkali substance, as a complication of radiation therapy, or as a complication of trauma (burns; food poisoning; severe infection; liver, kidney, or respiratory failure; major surgery).

- Chronic gastritis occurs in the presence of ulcers (benign or malignant), *Helicobacter pylori*, autoimmune disorders (pernicious anemia), poor diet (excessive caffeine, excessive alcohol intake), medications (alendronate, perindopril), and reflux of pancreatic secretions and bile into stomach.
- Manifestations include abdominal pain or discomfort (can be relieved by eating), headache, lethargy, nausea, anorexia, hiccuping (lasting a few hours to days), heartburn after eating, belching, sour taste in mouth, vomiting, bleeding, and hematemesis (vomiting of blood).
- Acute recovery typically occurs in 1 day, but can take 2 to 3 days. The client should eat a bland diet when able to tolerate food. IV fluid replacement therapy is indicated if the condition persists.
- When the condition occurs due to ingestion of strong acids or alkalis, dilution and neutralization of the causal agent is needed. Avoid lavage and emetics due to potential perforation and esophageal damage. Qs

CHRONIC MANAGEMENT: Modify diet, reduce and manage stress, avoid alcohol and NSAIDs. If condition is persistent, the provider will prescribe an H_2 receptor antagonist such as ranitidine. QEBP

NURSING INTERVENTIONS

- Suggest that the client avoid eating frequent meals and snacks, as they promote increased gastric acid secretion.
- Tell the client to avoid alcohol, cigarette smoking, aspirin and other nonsteroidal anti-inflammatory drugs (NSAIDs), coffee, black pepper, spicy foods, and caffeine.
- Monitor the client for vitamin deficiency, especially of vitamin B_{12}.

Peptic ulcer disease

- Peptic ulcer disease (PUD) is characterized by an erosion of the mucosal layer of the stomach or duodenum.
- This can be caused by a bacterial infection with *H. pylori* or the chronic use of NSAIDs (aspirin, ibuprofen).
- Some clients who have PUD do not experience manifestations. Others report dull, gnawing pain, burning sensation in the back or low midepigastric area, heartburn, constipation or diarrhea, sour taste in mouth, burping, nausea, vomiting, bloating, urea present in breath, and tarry stools. Eating can temporarily relieve pain. Anemia can occur due to blood loss.
- For PUD caused by *H. pylori*, the provider prescribes triple therapy (a combination of antibiotics and acid reducing medications) to be taken for 14 days.

NURSING INTERVENTIONS

- Advise the client to avoid eating frequent meals and snacks as they promote increased gastric acid secretion.
- Suggest that the client avoid coffee, alcohol, caffeine, aspirin and other NSAIDs, cigarette smoking, black pepper, and spicy foods.

Lactose intolerance

- Lactose intolerance results from an inadequate supply of lactase in the intestine, the enzyme that digests lactose.
- The enzyme that converts lactose into glucose, and galactose is absent or insufficient. Manifestations include distention, cramps, flatus, and osmotic diarrhea.

NURSING INTERVENTIONS

- Encourage clients to avoid or limit their intake of foods high in lactose (milk, cheese, ice cream, cream soups, sour cream, puddings, chocolate, coffee creamer).
- Suggest that the client ask the provider about the use of a lactase enzyme.
- Monitor the client for vitamin D deficiency and calcium.

Ileostomies and colostomies

An ostomy is a surgically created opening on the surface of the abdomen from either the end of the small intestine (ileostomy) or from the colon (colostomy).

- Fluid and electrolyte maintenance is the primary concern for clients who have ileostomies and colostomies.
- The colon absorbs large amounts of fluid, sodium, and potassium.
- Nutrition therapy begins with liquids only and is slowly advanced based upon client tolerance.

NURSING INTERVENTIONS

- Advise the client to consume a diet that is high in fluids and soluble fiber.
- Encourage the client to avoid foods that cause gas (beans, eggs, carbonated beverages), stomal blockage (nuts, raw carrots, popcorn), and foods that produce odor (eggs, fish, garlic).
- Encourage the client to increase his intake of calories and protein to promote healing of the stoma site.
- Provide emotional support to clients due to the risk of altered body image. Qpcc

Diverticulosis and diverticulitis

Diverticula are pouches protruding through the muscle of the intestinal wall, usually from increased intraluminal pressure. They occur anywhere in the colon, but usually in the sigmoid colon. Unless infection occurs, diverticula cause no problems.

- Diverticulosis is a condition characterized by the presence of diverticula.
- Diverticulitis is inflammation that occurs when fecal matter becomes trapped in the diverticula.
- Manifestations of diverticulitis include abdominal pain, nausea, vomiting, constipation or diarrhea, and fever, accompanied by chills and tachycardia.
- The client receives antibiotics, anticholinergics, and analgesics. Clients who have severe manifestations are admitted to the hospital and dehydration is treated with IV therapy. Opioid analgesics are administered for pain. Complications (peritonitis, bowel obstruction, abscess) can warrant surgical intervention.
- A high-fiber diet can prevent diverticulosis and diverticulitis by producing stools that are easily passed, thus decreasing pressure within the colon.

- During acute diverticulitis, a clear liquid diet is prescribed until inflammation decreases, then a high-fiber, low-fat diet is indicated.
- Instruct the client to avoid foods with seeds or husks (corn, popcorn, berries, tomatoes).
- Clients require instruction regarding diet adjustment based on the need for an acute intervention or preventive approach.

Inflammatory bowel disease (IBD)

- Crohn's disease (regional enteritis) and ulcerative colitis are chronic, inflammatory bowel diseases characterized by periods of exacerbation and remission.
- Manifestations include nausea, vomiting, abdominal cramps, fever, fatigue, anorexia, weight loss, steatorrhea, and low-grade fever.
- Nutrition therapy is focused on providing nutrients in forms that the client can tolerate.
- Generally, diets are low in fiber to minimize bowel stimulation.
- A low-residue, high-protein, high-calorie diet with vitamin and mineral supplementation is prescribed. Fluid and electrolyte imbalances are corrected with IV fluids or oral replacement fluids.
- Teach clients to avoid intake of substances that cause or exacerbate diarrhea, and to avoid nicotine.
- Total parenteral nutrition (TPN) is indicated for clients who are severely ill during the acute phase of the illness.

ADDITIONAL THERAPY

- Sedatives
- Antidiarrheal and antiperistaltic agents
- Aminosalicylate medications and corticosteroids to reduce inflammation
- Immunomodulators to alter the immune response and prevent relapse
- Surgery when other treatments are not effective

Cholecystitis

- Cholecystitis is characterized by inflammation of the gallbladder.
- The gallbladder stores and releases bile that aids in the digestion of fats.
- Manifestations include pain, tenderness, and rigidity in upper right abdomen. Pain can radiate to the right shoulder or midsternal area. Nausea, vomiting, and anorexia also can occur. If the gallbladder becomes filled with pus or becomes gangrenous, perforation can result.
- In clients who have large stones or inability to control the condition with diet modifications, surgery is required.
- Pancreatitis and liver involvement can result from uncontrolled cholecystitis.
- Fat intake should be limited to reduce stimulation of the gallbladder.
- Other foods that can cause problems include coffee, broccoli, cauliflower, Brussels sprouts, cabbage, onions, legumes, and highly seasoned foods.
- The diet is individualized to the client's needs and tolerance.

Pancreatitis

- Pancreatitis is an inflammation of the pancreas.
- The pancreas is responsible for secreting enzymes needed to digest fats, carbohydrates, and proteins.
- Nutritional therapy for acute pancreatitis involves reducing pancreatic stimulation. The client is prescribed nothing by mouth (NPO), and a nasogastric tube is inserted to suction gastric contents.
- TPN can be used until oral intake is resumed.
- Nutritional therapy for chronic pancreatitis usually includes a low-fat, high-protein, and high-carbohydrate diet. It can include providing supplements of vitamin C and B-complex vitamins.

Liver disease

- The liver is involved in the metabolism of most nutrients.
- Disorders affecting the liver include cirrhosis, hepatitis, and cancer.
- Malnutrition is common with liver disease.
- Protein needs are increased to promote a positive nitrogen balance and prevent a breakdown of the body's protein stores.
- Carbohydrates are generally not restricted, as they are an important source of calories.
- Caloric requirements might need to be increased based on an evaluation of the client's stage of disease, weight, and general health status.
- Multivitamins (especially vitamins B, C, and K) and mineral supplements might be necessary.
- Alcohol, nicotine, and caffeine should be eliminated.

Celiac disease QPCC

- Celiac disease is also known as gluten-sensitive enteropathy, celiac sprue, and gluten intolerance.
- It is a chronic, inherited, genetic disorder with autoimmune characteristics. Clients who have celiac disease are unable to digest the protein gluten. They lack the digestive enzyme DPP-IV, which is required to break down the gluten into molecules small enough to be used by the body. In celiac disease, gluten is broken down into peptide strands instead of molecules. The body is not able to metabolize the peptides. If untreated, the client will suffer destruction of the villa and the walls of the small intestine. Celiac disease can go undiagnosed in both children and adults.
- Manifestations vary widely. Children who have celiac disease have diarrhea, steatorrhea, anemia, abdominal distention, impaired growth, lack of appetite, and fatigue. Typical manifestations in adults include diarrhea, abdominal pain, bloating, anemia, steatorrhea, and osteomalacia.
- Treatment for celiac disease is limited to avoiding gluten. However, eliminating gluten, which is found in wheat, rye and barley, is difficult because it is found in many prepared foods. Clients must read food labels carefully in order to adhere to a gluten-free diet. Some gluten-free products are unappealing to clients, and many are more expensive than other products. Prognosis is good for clients who adhere to a gluten-free diet.

NURSING INTERVENTIONS

- Encourage clients to eat foods that are gluten-free: milk, cheese, rice, corn, eggs, potatoes, fruits, vegetables, fresh meats and fish, dried beans.
- Remind clients to read labels on processed products. Gravy mixes, sauces, cold cuts, soups, and many other products have gluten as an ingredient. Advise clients to read labels and research nonfood products (e.g., lipstick, communion wafers, vitamin supplements), which also can have gluten as an ingredient.

Bariatric surgery

- Considered the most effective treatment for severe obesity.
- Benefits include reduction of diabetes mellitus, hypertension, dyslipidemia, and mortality rates as well as improved quality of life.
- **Adjustable gastric banding:** restricts stomach capacity to 15-30mL with an inflatable band that encircles the uppermost portion of the stomach, similar to a "belt" to create an outlet that can be adjusted as needed.
  - Instruct client that diet will gradually increase from liquids to pureed to soft foods.
  - Instruct client on the importance of chewing foods thoroughly, slowly and in small amounts.
- **Roux-en-Y gastric bypass:** Ingested food bypasses 95% of the stomach, the duodenum, and a small portion of the proximal jejunum. Weight loss is achieved through malabsorption and dumping syndrome and the altering of the hormone ghrelin which decreases hunger.
  - Possible postoperative complications include anastomotic leaks, internal hernias, GI bleeding, stomal stenosis, gallstones.
  - Micronutrient deficiencies are common long term.
- **Sleeve gastrectomy** is a newer procedure that can also be performed. A longitudinal portion of the stomach is removed to create a "sleeve" effect. Reduces the hormone ghrelin which decreases hunger.
- Bariatric surgery works best in combination with diet and lifestyle changes. Nutritional counseling is essential.
- Instruct client that dramatic changes in food intake and regular physical activity will be necessary for successful long-term weight control.

Application Exercises

1. A nurse is teaching a client who is recovering from pancreatitis about following a low-fat diet. Which of the following foods should the nurse recommend? ? (Select all that apply.)

   A. Ribeye steak

   B. Oatmeal

   C. Ice cream

   D. Canned peaches

   E. Pretzels

2. A nurse is teaching a client who has constipation about a high-fiber, low-fat diet. Which of the following food choices by the client indicates understanding of the teaching?

   A. Peanut butter

   B. Peeled apples

   C. Hardboiled egg

   D. Brown rice

3. A nurse is assessing a client who is postoperative from a gastric bypass and who just finished eating a meal. Which of the following findings are manifestations of dumping syndrome? (Select all that apply.)

   A. Bradycardia

   B. Dizziness

   C. Dry skin

   D. Hypotension

   E. Diarrhea

4. A nurse is collecting data from a client who has peptic ulcer disease (PUD). Which of the following findings should the nurse expect? (Select all that apply.)

   A. Steatorrhea

   B. Anemia

   C. Tarry stools

   D. Epigastric pain

   E. Swollen lymph nodes

5. A nurse is instructing a client who has celiac disease about foods to avoid. Which of the following foods should the nurse include in the teaching?

   A. Potatoes

   B. Graham crackers

   C. Wild rice

   D. Canned pears

PRACTICE Active Learning Scenario

A nurse is providing instructions to the parent of a child who has lactose intolerance. What should the nurse include in the teaching? Use the ATI Active Learning Template: System Disorder to complete this item.

CLIENT EDUCATION
- Describe the underlying cause of lactose intolerance.
- Identify two manifestations of lactose intolerance.
- Identify three foods the child should limit or eliminate from his diet.

Application Exercises Key

1. A. Ribeye steak is not a low-fat food source.

    B. **CORRECT:** Oatmeal is a source of easily digested carbohydrate that is low in fat.

    C. Ice cream is not a low-fat food source.

    D. **CORRECT:** Canned peaches are a source of easily digested carbohydrate that is low in fat.

    E. **CORRECT:** Pretzels are a source of easily digested carbohydrate that is low in fat.

    Ⓝ *NCLEX® Connection: Basic Care and Comfort, Nutrition and Oral Hydration*

2. A. Peanut butter is high in fat. This choice indicates that the client does not understand the teaching.

    B. Unpeeled fruit is a better source of fiber. This choice indicates that the client does not understand the teaching.

    C. Egg yolk is high in fat. This choice indicates that the client does not understand the teaching.

    D. **CORRECT:** Brown rice is a good source of fiber and is low in fat. This choice indicates that the client understands the teaching.

    Ⓝ *NCLEX® Connection: Basic Care and Comfort, Elimination*

3. A. When a portion of the stomach is no longer available to serve as a reservoir, a large amount of food is rapidly dumped into the small intestine, and fluid shifts from general circulation into the intestine. Tachycardia occurs due to a decrease in circulating volume.

    B. **CORRECT:** When a portion of the stomach is no longer available to serve as a reservoir, a large amount of food is rapidly dumped into the small intestine, and fluid shifts from general circulation into the intestine. Dizziness occurs due to a decrease in circulating volume.

    C. Sweating, not dry skin, is a clinical manifestation of dumping syndrome.

    D. **CORRECT:** When a portion of the stomach is no longer available to serve as a reservoir, a large amount of food is rapidly dumped into the small intestine, and fluid shifts from general circulation into the intestine. Hypotension occurs due to a decrease in circulating volume.

    E. **CORRECT:** When a portion of the stomach is no longer available to serve as a reservoir, a large amount of food is rapidly dumped into the small intestine, which causes increased peristalsis, and diarrhea occurs.

    Ⓝ *NCLEX® Connection: Basic Care and Comfort, Elimination*

4. A. Steatorrhea is a clinical finding in the presence celiac disease.

    B. **CORRECT:** Iron deficiency anemia due to blood loss is a clinical finding of PUD.

    C. **CORRECT:** Tarry stools due to intestinal bleeding is a clinical finding of PUD.

    D. **CORRECT:** Epigastric pain described as a gnawing or burning sensation is a clinical manifestation of PUD.

    E. Swollen lymph nodes are a clinical manifestation of many conditions and infections, but not of PUD.

    Ⓝ *NCLEX® Connection: Basic Care and Comfort, Elimination*

5. A. Potatoes are gluten-free and a good choice for a client who has celiac disease.

    B. **CORRECT:** Graham crackers are made from wheat flour. A client who has celiac disease should avoid products that are made from wheat flour.

    C. Wild rice is gluten-free and a good choice for a client who has celiac disease.

    D. Fruits and vegetables without a sauce are gluten-free and are good choices for a client who has celiac disease.

    Ⓝ *NCLEX® Connection: Basic Care and Comfort, Nutrition and Oral Hydration*

PRACTICE Answer

Using the ATI Active Learning Template: System Disorder

CLIENT EDUCATION

- The underlying cause of lactose intolerance. Lactose intolerance is due to an inadequate level of lactase. The enzyme that converts lactose into glucose and galactose is absent or insufficient.

- Manifestations
  - Abdominal distension
  - Cramps
  - Flatus
  - Diarrhea

- Foods to limit or avoid include milk, cheese, ice cream, cream soups, puddings, and chocolate.

Ⓝ *NCLEX® Connection: Physiological Adaptation, Illness Management*

CHAPTER 14

CHAPTER 14 *Renal Disorders*

Nurses must understand nutritional needs of clients who have renal disorders. It is important to explore dietary needs with the client and recommend modifications related to the disease process. Understanding the role of primary and secondary prevention is essential to successful treatment.

Nutritional considerations for the following kidney disorders covered in this chapter are chronic kidney disease (stage 1 to 4), end-stage kidney disease (stage 5), acute kidney injury, nephrotic syndrome, and nephrolithiasis (kidney stones).

The kidneys have two primary functions: maintaining blood volume and excreting waste products. Other functions include the regulation of acid-base balance, blood pressure, calcium and phosphorous metabolism, and red blood cell production. Kidney damage and/or loss of kidney function have profound effects on the client's nutritional state. Urea is a waste by-product of protein metabolism, and urea levels rise with kidney disease. Monitoring protein intake is critical.

Short-term kidney disease requires nutritional support for healing rather than dietary restrictions. Dietary recommendations are dependent upon the stage of kidney disease.

ASSESSMENT/DATA COLLECTION

Chronic kidney disease (stages 1 to 4) is distinguished by an increase in serum creatinine. Manifestations include fatigue, back pain, and appetite changes.

End-stage kidney disease (ESKD) manifestations include fatigue, decreased alertness, anemia, decreased urination, headache, and weight loss.

Acute kidney injury (AKI) manifestations include a decrease in urination, decreased sensation in the extremities, swelling of the lower extremities, and flank pain. It is characterized by rising blood levels of urea and other nitrogenous wastes.

Nephrotic syndrome's most pronounced manifestations are edema and high proteinuria. Other manifestations include hypoalbuminemia, hyperlipidemia, and blood hypercoagulation.

Kidney stones are characterized by sudden, intense pain that is typically located in the flank and is unrelieved by position changes as the stone moves out of the kidney pelvis and down the ureter. Diaphoresis, nausea, and vomiting are common, and there can be blood in the urine. The majority of kidney stones are made of calcium oxalate.

NUTRITIONAL GUIDELINES AND NURSING INTERVENTIONS

General renal considerations

- Monitor kidney parameters for clients who have renal disorders.
  - Nurses should monitor weight daily or as prescribed. Weight is an indicator of fluid status, which is a primary concern. Q͏EBP
  - Monitor fluid intake, and encourage compliance with fluid restrictions.
  - Nurses should monitor urine output. Placement of an indwelling urinary catheter might be necessary for accurate measurement.
  - Monitor for manifestations of constipation. Fluid restrictions predispose clients to constipation.
- Explain why dietary changes are necessary. Alterations in the intake of protein, calories, sodium, potassium, phosphorus, and other vitamins are required.
- Provide support for the client and family.

Chronic kidney disease (stages 1 to 4)

- CKD is a progressively worsening disorder that is categorized in stages.
  - Stage 1: at risk for CKD
  - Stage 2: mild CKD
  - Stage 3: moderate CKD
  - Stage 4: severe CKD
- Stages 1 to 4 are predialysis and characterized by increasing serum creatinine levels and a decreasing glomerular filtration rate (GFR).
- The leading causes of CKD are diabetes mellitus and hypertension. Other causes include contrast dye, certain medications, cardiovascular disease, obesity, hypercholesterolemia, recurrent urinary tract infections, HIV, immunologic disease, and family history.
- More common in African Americans, Native Americans, and Hispanics.

THERAPEUTIC NUTRITION

- Goals of nutritional therapy
  - Slow the progression of CKD.
  - Control blood glucose and hypertension.
  - Help preserve remaining kidney function by limiting the intake of protein and phosphorus.
- Restricting phosphorus intake slows the progression of kidney disease. High levels of phosphorus contribute to calcium and phosphorus deposits in the kidneys.
- Protein restriction is essential for clients who have stage 1-4 CKD.
  - Slows the progression of kidney disease.
  - Too little protein results in the breakdown of body protein. Carefully determine protein intake.

DIETARY RECOMMENDATIONS

- Restrict sodium intake to maintain blood pressure.
- Restrict potassium intake to prevent hyperkalemia.
- The recommended daily protein intake is 0.8 to 1.0 g/kg/day of ideal body weight.
  - Protein restrictions are decreased as the disease progresses to ESKD, and to decrease the workload on the kidneys.
  - High biologic value proteins are recommended for clients who have CKD to prevent catabolism of muscle tissue. These proteins include eggs, meats, poultry, game, fish, soy, and dairy products.
- Limit meat intake to 5 to 6 oz/day for most men and 4 oz/day for most women.
- Limit dairy products to ½ cup per day.
- Limit high-phosphorus foods (peanut butter, dried peas and beans, bran, cola, chocolate, beer, some whole grains) to one serving or less per day.
- Caution clients to use vitamin and mineral supplements only when recommended by a provider. Avoid high protein sports drinks, energy drinks, or meal supplements. Avoid herbal supplements that can affect bleeding time and blood pressure. Qs

End-stage kidney disease

ESKD, or Stage 5 CKD, occurs when the GFR is less than 15 mL/min, the serum creatinine level steadily rises, or dialysis or transplantation is necessary.

THERAPEUTIC NUTRITION

- The goal of nutritional therapy is to maintain appropriate fluid status, blood pressure, and blood chemistries.
  - A high-protein, low-phosphorus, low-potassium, low-sodium (2 to 4 g/day), fluid-restricted diet is recommended.
  - Once dialysis begins, protein intake should increase because some protein is lost during dialysis. The amount of protein increase will depend on whether hemodialysis or peritoneal dialysis is being performed.
  - Monitor vitamin D and calcium, and replace as needed.
- Monitor potassium level and replace as needed. Sodium and fluid allowances are determined by blood pressure, weight, serum electrolyte findings, and urine output.
- Achieving a well-balanced diet based on the above guidelines is difficult. The National Renal Diet provides clients with a list of food choices.
- Protein needs increase once dialysis has begun as protein and amino acids are lost in the dialysate.
  - Fifty percent of protein intake should come from biologic sources (eggs, milk, meat, fish, poultry, soy).
  - Consume adequate calories (35 kcal/kg of body weight) to maintain body protein stores.
- Restrict phosphorus.
  - A high protein requirement leads to an increase in phosphorus intake.
  - Foods high in phosphorus are milk products, beef liver, chocolate, nuts, and legumes.
  - Phosphate binders (e.g., calcium carbonate, calcium acetate) are taken with all meals and snacks.
- Vitamin D deficiency occurs as the kidneys are unable to convert vitamin D to its active form.
  - This alters the metabolism of calcium, phosphorus, and magnesium, leading to hyperphosphatemia, hypocalcemia, and hypermagnesemia.
  - Calcium supplements will likely be required because foods high in phosphorus (which are restricted) are also high in calcium.

Acute kidney injury

AKI is an abrupt, rapid decline in kidney function caused by trauma, sepsis, poor perfusion, or medications, and usually is reversible. AKI can cause hyponatremia, hyperkalemia, hypocalcemia, and hyperphosphatemia. Fluid overload leading to pulmonary edema is a complication of AKI.

THERAPEUTIC NUTRITION

- Diet therapy for AKI is dependent upon the phase of AKI and its underlying cause. Protein, calories, fluids, potassium, and sodium need to be individualized according to the three phases of AKI (oliguric, diuretic, and recovery phase), and adjusted as needed and if the client is receiving dialysis.
- Recommendation is to consume 25 to 50 cal/kg of body weight to maintain energy and demands of stress.
- Simple carbohydrates, fats, oils, and low-protein starches are included in the diet. Provide nonprotein calories in an adequate amount to maintain the client's weight.
- Protein intake can increase to 1 to 1.5 g/kg if the client is receiving dialysis, compared to 0.6 g/kg (40 g/day) for nondialysis clients.
- Potassium and sodium are dependent on urine output, serum values, and if the client is receiving dialysis.
  - Potassium is restricted to 60 to 70 mEq/day when on dialysis.
  - Sodium is restricted to 1 to 3 g/day if not receiving dialysis, and 1 to 4 g/day if receiving dialysis, which also depends on the phase.
  - Calcium requirements are of less than 2,000 mg daily if on hemodialysis or peritoneal dialysis.
- Fluids are restricted to the client's daily urine output plus 500 mL during the oliguric phase. Fluid needs are increased during the diuretic phase.

Nephrotic syndrome

- Nephrotic syndrome results in the increased excretion of serum proteins into the urine, resulting in hypoalbuminemia, edema, hyperlipidemia, and blood hypercoagulation. Prolonged protein loss leads to protein malnutrition, anemia, and vitamin D deficiency.
- Diabetes mellitus, kidney damage due to medications or chemicals, autoimmune disorders, and infections can cause nephrotic syndrome.

THERAPEUTIC NUTRITION

- Nutritional therapy goals include minimizing edema, replacing lost nutrients, minimizing kidney damage, controlling hypertension, and preventing protein malnutrition that can lead to muscle catabolism.
- Dietary recommendations indicate sufficient protein and low sodium intake.
  - Adequate amount of protein intake is 0.7 to 0.8 g/kg/day.
  - Soy-based proteins can decrease protein losses and lower serum lipid levels.
  - Low-sodium diet of 2,000 to 3,000 mg/day can help control edema and hypertension.
  - Carbohydrates should provide the majority of the client's daily calories.
  - Foods high in trans fats and cholesterol are limited, and total fat should be less than 30% of the daily diet.
  - Provide a multiple vitamin supplement to replace loss of vitamins with protein excretion.

Nephrolithiasis

- The most common type of kidney stone is made of calcium oxalate.
- Contributing factors include inadequate fluid intake, elevated urine pH, and excess excretion through the kidneys of oxalate, calcium, and uric acid.
- Kidney stone formation is more influenced by the amount of oxalate in the client's system than calcium. A client who has an ileostomy has an increased risk of kidney stones.

PREVENTATIVE NUTRITION: Excessive intake of protein, sodium, calcium, and oxalates (rhubarb, spinach, beets) can increase the risk of stone formation.

THERAPEUTIC NUTRITION

- Increasing fluid consumption is the primary intervention for the treatment and prevention of kidney stones. Daily fluid intake should be at least 1,500 mL to 3,000 mL. At least 8 to 12 oz (240 to 360 mL) of fluid, preferably water, should be consumed before bedtime because urine becomes more concentrated at night.
- Recommendation for calcium oxalate stone formation is to limit animal protein, excess sodium, alcohol, and caffeine use. Low potassium can contribute to calcium stone formation.
- Foods high in oxalates include spinach, rhubarb, beets, nuts, chocolate, tea, wheat bran, and strawberries, and should be limited in the diet. Avoid megadoses of vitamin C, which increase the amount of oxalate excreted.
- Recommendation for prevention of uric acid stones is to limit foods high in purines, which include lean meats, organ meats, whole grains, and legumes.

Application Exercises

1. A nurse is planning care for a client who has ESKD. Which of the following should the nurse include in the plan of care? (Select all that apply.)

    A. Monitor the client's weight daily.

    B. Encourage the client to comply with fluid restrictions.

    C. Evaluate intake and output.

    D. Instruct the client on restricting calories from carbohydrates.

    E. Monitor for constipation.

2. A nurse is teaching a client who has stage 2 chronic kidney disease about dietary management. Which of the following information should the nurse include in the instructions?

    A. Restrict protein intake.

    B. Maintain a high-phosphorus diet.

    C. Increase intake of foods high in potassium.

    D. Limit dairy products to 1 cup/day.

3. A nurse is teaching a client about protein needs when on dialysis. Which of the following instructions should the nurse include in the teaching? (Select all that apply.)

    A. Consume 35 kcal/kg of body weight to maintain body protein stores.

    B. Take phosphate binders when eating protein-rich foods.

    C. Increase biologic sources of protein, such as eggs, milk, and soy.

    D. Increase protein intake by 50% of the recommended dietary allowance (RDA).

    E. Consume daily protein intake in the morning.

4. A nurse is teaching about diet restrictions to a client who has acute kidney injury and is on hemodialysis. Which of the following recommendations should the nurse include in the teaching?

    A. Limit calcium intake to 2,500 mg/day.

    B. Decrease total fat intake to 45% of daily calories.

    C. Decrease potassium intake to 65 mEq/day.

    D. Limit sodium intake to 4.5 g/day.

5. A nurse is completing discharge teaching about diet and fluid restrictions to a client who has a calcium oxalate-based kidney stone. Which of the following instructions should the nurse include in the teaching?

    A. Reduce intake of spinach.

    B. Decrease broccoli intake.

    C. Increase intake of vitamin C supplements.

    D. Limit consumption of purine substances.

PRACTICE Active Learning Scenario

A nurse is reviewing teaching for a client who has nephrotic syndrome. What information should the nurse include? Use the ATI Active Learning Template: System Disorder to complete this item.

ALTERATION IN HEALTH (DIAGNOSIS)

COMPLICATIONS: List three.

CLIENT EDUCATION: Include five teaching points.

Application Exercises Key

1. A. **CORRECT:** Monitoring the client's daily weight assists in determining fluid retention.

   B. **CORRECT:** Implementing fluid restriction for a client helps to slow fluid retention.

   C. **CORRECT:** Evaluating I&O helps to determine if there is an increase in fluid retention.

   D. Carbohydrates are not restricted for a client who has ESKD.

   E. **CORRECT:** Constipation often occurs as a result of fluid restrictions.

   Ⓝ *NCLEX® Connection: Basic Care and Comfort, Nutrition and Oral Hydration*

2. A. **CORRECT:** Restricting protein intake decreases the risk for proteinuria and decreases the workload on the kidney.

   B. A diet high in phosphorus is not recommended because it can contribute to calcium and phosphorus deposits on the kidney.

   C. Eating foods low in potassium is recommended because hyperkalemia occurs with kidney disease.

   D. Dairy products are a protein and sodium source, and are limited to 0.5 cup/day.

   Ⓝ *NCLEX® Connection: Basic Care and Comfort, Nutrition and Oral Hydration*

3. A. **CORRECT:** To maintain protein stores, the client should consume 35 cal/kg of body weight.

   B. **CORRECT:** Protein consumption increases phosphorus intake. Phosphate binders are recommended with meals.

   C. **CORRECT:** Protein intake should include biologic sources of protein to include eggs, milk, meat, fish, poultry, and soy.

   D. **CORRECT:** The recommended protein intake for a client on dialysis is 50% greater than the RDA because amino acids are lost in the dialysate.

   E. The client should spread protein intake throughout the day to prevent excessive intake of phosphorous and potassium.

   Ⓝ *NCLEX® Connection: Basic Care and Comfort, Nutrition and Oral Hydration*

4. A. The client receiving hemodialysis should limit calcium intake to less than 2,000 mg/day.

   B. The client should limit total fat intake to 35% of daily calories.

   C. **CORRECT:** The client should limit potassium intake to 60 to 70 mEq/day.

   D. The client should limit sodium intake to 1 to 4 g/day when receiving dialysis.

   Ⓝ *NCLEX® Connection: Basic Care and Comfort, Nutrition and Oral Hydration*

5. A. **CORRECT:** The client should reduce intake of foods high in oxalate, such as spinach, which can cause calcium stone formation.

   B. Broccoli is high in calcium but does not cause calcium stone formation and is not restricted in the diet.

   C. Large doses of vitamin C supplements can cause calcium stone formation.

   D. Foods that contain purine, such as organ meats and red wine, cause uric acid stone formation.

   Ⓝ *NCLEX® Connection: Health Promotion and Maintenance, Health Promotion/Disease Prevention*

PRACTICE Answer

Using the ATI Active Learning Template: System Disorder

ALTERATION IN HEALTH (DIAGNOSIS): Nephrotic syndrome is a renal disorder in which there is increased excretion of serum proteins into the urine.

COMPLICATIONS

- Hypoalbuminemia
- Proteinuria
- Edema
- Hyperlipidemia
- Malnutrition
- Anemia

CLIENT EDUCATION

- Increase protein intake to prevent catabolism of muscle tissue.
- Limit sodium intake to control edema and hypertension.
- Consume foods low in trans fats and cholesterol.
- Consume foods high in carbohydrates to increase calorie intake.
- Take a vitamin supplement to replace vitamin loss that occurs with protein excretion.

Ⓝ *NCLEX® Connection: Physiological Adaptation, Illness Management*

UNIT 3   ALTERATIONS IN NUTRITION

CHAPTER 15 *Diabetes Mellitus*

Nurses must be aware of nutritional needs for clients who have diabetes mellitus. It is important for the nurse to explore dietary needs with the client and recommend modifications related to the disease process. Understanding the role of primary and secondary prevention is essential to successful management.

Diabetes mellitus inhibits the body's production and/or use of insulin. This results in greater-than-normal glucose levels and can result in health complications including heart disease, blindness, kidney failure, and deterioration or decreased function of nerves.

Glucose is the body's primary source of energy, and insulin is needed to assist the body in the breakdown of glucose to a form that is used for energy. The goal of management is to assist the client in making lifestyle changes and nutritional choices necessary to control blood glucose levels. Achieving proper nutrition and meeting specific dietary needs is essential in controlling the effects of diabetes mellitus. Blood glucose levels are used to diagnose diabetes.

TYPES OF DIABETES MELLITUS

Type 1 diabetes mellitus

- Autoimmune disease triggered by genetic links or a viral infection.
- Damage to or destruction of beta cells of the pancreas results in an absence of insulin production.
- Usually occurs in individuals under the age of 30 whose weight is within ideal healthy body weight.

RISK FACTORS
- Relative who has diabetes mellitus
- History of viral infections, such as coxsackievirus, and mumps

Type 2 diabetes mellitus

- Results from genetic and environmental factors
- Characterized by altered patterns of insulin secretion and decreased cellular uptake of glucose (insulin resistance)

RISK FACTORS
- Age older than 45 years
- Hypertension
- Hyperlipidemia
- African American, Latino, Native American, Asian American, and Pacific Islander ethnic groups
- Obesity and sedentary lifestyle
- Relative who has diabetes mellitus

Gestational diabetes mellitus (GDM)

- Glucose intolerance that is recognized during pregnancy.
- Usually occurs during the second and third trimesters.
- Occurs only during pregnancy and typically resolves after delivery.
- Characterized by increased insulin resistance caused by secretion of placental hormones, and increased insulin antagonists.
- Many women who have GDM develop type 2 diabetes mellitus later in life.
- Blood glucose control is important in preventing damage to the fetus of women who are pregnant and who have GDM or pre-existing diabetes mellitus.

INCREASES THE RISK FOR
- Preeclampsia
- Cesarean delivery
- Large newborn birth weight
- Infant hyperglycemia
- Infant death
- Maternal hypertension and diabetes mellitus after pregnancy

ASSESSMENT/DATA COLLECTION

Hypoglycemia is a blood glucose level below the expected reference range. It results from taking too much insulin, inadequate food intake, delayed or skipped meals, extra physical activity, or consumption of alcohol without food.

- Blood glucose of 70 mg/dL or less requires immediate action.
- Manifestations include mild shakiness, mental confusion, sweating, palpitations, headache, lack of coordination, blurred vision, seizures, and coma.

Hyperglycemia is a blood glucose level above the expected reference range. It results from an imbalance with food, medication, and activity, combined with an inadequate amount of insulin production or cells that are insulin-resistant.

- Infection, other illness, and stress can cause a rise in blood glucose.
- Manifestations include blood glucose greater than 200 mg/dL, ketones in urine, polydipsia (excessive thirst), polyuria (excessive urination), polyphagia (excess hunger and eating), hyperventilation (Kussmaul respirations), dehydration, fruity odor to the breath, headache, inability to concentrate, decreased levels of consciousness, and seizures leading to coma.

NUTRITIONAL GUIDELINES AND NURSING INTERVENTIONS

Hypoglycemia

- Clients who have hypoglycemia should take 10 to 20 g of a readily absorbable carbohydrate. Qs
  - Two or three glucose tablets (5 g each)
  - Six to ten hard candies
  - ½ cup (4 oz) juice or regular soda
  - 1 tbsp honey or 4 tsp sugar
- Retest the blood glucose in 15 min. If it is less than 70 mg/dL, repeat the above steps. Once levels stabilize, have the client take an additional carbohydrate and protein snack or small meal, depending on the severity of the hypoglycemic episode and whether the next meal is more than 1 hr away.

Hyperglycemia

- Clients who have hyperglycemia should do the following.
  - Immediately consult a provider, or go to the emergency department.
  - Take medication if forgotten.
  - Consider modifications to insulin or oral diabetic medications.
- Long-term implications of untreated or inadequately treated hyperglycemia include blindness, kidney failure, dyslipidemia, hypertension, neuropathy, microvascular and macrovascular disease, and limb amputation.
- The Somogyi phenomenon is morning hyperglycemia in response to overnight hypoglycemia. Providing a bedtime snack and appropriate insulin dose prevents this phenomenon.
- The dawn phenomenon is an elevation of blood glucose around 0500 to 0600. It results from an overnight release of growth hormone, and is treated by increasing the amount of insulin provided during the overnight hours.

GENERAL NUTRITIONAL GUIDELINES

- Coronary heart disease (CHD) is a frequent cause of death among clients who have diabetes. Clients who have diabetes are encouraged to follow a diet that is high in fiber and low in saturated fat, trans fat, and cholesterol.
- Dietary intake should be individualized according to the client's food intake, need for weight management, and lipid and glucose patterns.
  - **Carbohydrates**
    - Encourage the client to consume carbohydrates found in grains, fruits, legumes, and milk. Limit simple carbohydrates, which include refined grains and sugars.
    - Carbohydrates should include a minimum of 130 g/day for healthy brain function.
    - Carbohydrates should be 45% to 65% of total daily caloric intake.
  - **Fats**
    - Saturated fat should account for less than 7% of total calories.
    - Trans fatty acid recommendation is less than 1% of total daily caloric intake. Limit fried foods and bakery products, which contain high quantities of trans fatty acid from preparation with hydrogenated oils.
    - Cholesterol is restricted to 200 to 300 mg/day.
    - Polyunsaturated fatty acids are found in fish. Two or more servings per week are recommended.
  - **Fiber**
    - Promote fiber intake (beans, vegetables, oats, whole grains) to improve carbohydrate metabolism and lower cholesterol.
    - Recommendation for fiber intake includes at least 14 g per 1,000 calories.
  - **Protein:** Protein from meats, eggs, fish, nuts, beans, and soy products should comprise 15% to 20% of total caloric intake. Reduce protein intake if needed in clients who have diabetes and kidney failure.
- Encourage clients who have diabetes mellitus to eliminate all tobacco use due to the increased risk of cardiovascular disease.
- Recommended maximum daily alcohol consumption for a client who has well-controlled diabetes is one alcoholic beverage for women or two for men.
  - To avoid hypoglycemia, the client should consume alcohol with a meal or immediately after a meal.
  - Alcohol is not recommended for a client who has hyperlipidemia.
  - Alcoholic beverages should not replace food intake.
- Vitamin and mineral requirements are unchanged for clients who have diabetes. Supplements are recommended for identified deficiencies. Deficiencies in magnesium and potassium can aggravate glucose intolerance.
- Artificial sweeteners are acceptable. Saccharin crosses the placenta and should be avoided during pregnancy. Sucrose (table sugar) can be included in a diabetic diet as long as adequate insulin or other agents are provided to cover the sugar intake.
- Cultural and personal preferences should be considered in planning food intake. Qpcc

- According to the American Diabetes Association and the American Dietetic Association, daily nutritional requirements are based on the needs of each client. Qᴘᴄᴄ
  - The dietitian works with the client to develop meal planning that meets the client's needs based on healthy food choices.
  - The goal of therapy is to maintain blood glucose levels as close to the expected reference range as possible.
  - The dietitian instructs the client on various dietary methods, including exchange list and carbohydrate counting.
- Using the exchange list as a guide for meal planning allows for the incorporation of three basic food groups: protein, carbohydrates, and fats.
  - This dietary regimen assists the client in maintaining a blood glucose level within a target range.
  - Each client has a recommended amount of daily exchanges within each group based on the client's needs.
- Carbohydrate counting focuses on counting total grams of carbohydrates in each food item.
  - Each client is prescribed a number of grams of carbohydrates for each meal and daily snacks.
  - The dietitian determines the needs of the individual and provides instructions for reading food labels and counting carbohydrate amounts in food selections.
  - Clients can exchange carbohydrates as long as the portion size remains consistent.

OTHER NURSING INTERVENTIONS

- Encourage exercise. Closely monitor blood glucose and medication dosages.
- Encourage weight loss. It is important for clients who have type 2 diabetes mellitus as it can decrease insulin resistance, improve glucose and lipid levels, and lower blood pressure.
- Encourage clients to perform self-monitoring of blood glucose.
  - Strict control of glucose can reduce or postpone complications (retinopathy, nephropathy, neuropathy).
  - Teach proper calibration and use of the self-monitoring of blood glucose, record keeping, and reporting of levels to health care provider.
- Clients should receive regular evaluations from the provider.
- Client education and support is provided for the following.
  - Self-monitoring of blood glucose
  - Dietary and activity recommendations
  - Manifestations and treatment of hypoglycemia and hyperglycemia, to include the importance of taking medications as prescribed
  - Long-term complications of diabetes
  - Psychological implications
  - Community organizations and support groups whose focus is diabetes
- Children who have diabetes require parental support, guidance, and participation. Dietary intake must provide for proper growth and development.

Application Exercises

1. A nurse is providing information to a client who has a new diagnosis of type 1 diabetes mellitus. Which of the following information should the nurse include? (Select all that apply.)

    A. A viral infection can trigger the onset of type 1 diabetes mellitus.

    B. Alpha cells in the pancreas are damaged in type 1 diabetes mellitus.

    C. Type 1 diabetes mellitus usually occurs before age 30.

    D. Type 1 diabetes mellitus is treated with oral antiglycemic medications.

    E. Regular exercise can reduce insulin requirements in type 1 diabetes mellitus.

2. A nurse is assessing a client who is has hypoglycemia. Which of the following findings should the nurse expect?

    A. Fruity breath odor

    B. Diaphoresis

    C. Ketones in urine

    D. Polyuria

3. A nurse is caring for a client who has diabetes mellitus and is shaky and weak. Which of the following actions should the nurse take?

    A. Provide subcutaneous insulin for the client.

    B. Offer the client 120 mL (4 oz) fruit juice.

    C. Give the client IV potassium.

    D. Administer IV sodium bicarbonate.

4. A nurse is reinforcing dietary teaching to a client who has type 2 diabetes mellitus. Which of the following instructions should the nurse include in the teaching? (Select all that apply.)

    A. Carbohydrates should comprise 55% of daily caloric intake.

    B. Use hydrogenated oils for cooking.

    C. You can add table sugar to cereals.

    D. You can drink one alcoholic beverage with a meal.

    E. Use the same portion sizes to exchange carbohydrates.

5. A nurse is planning to create dietary guidelines for a client who has type 2 diabetes mellitus. Which of the following information should the nurse incorporate in the dietary plan? (Select all that apply.)

    A. Weight management

    B. Lipid profile

    C. Cultural needs

    D. Sleep patterns

    E. Personal preferences

PRACTICE Active Learning Scenario

A nurse is reviewing the discharge plan for a client who has type 1 diabetes mellitus. How should the nurse use interprofessional care in the plan? Use the ATI Active Learning Template: System Disorder to complete this item.

INTERPROFESSIONAL CARE: Describe the role of another member of the health care team.

CLIENT EDUCATION: Describe three teaching points offered by this member of the health team.

Application Exercises Key

1. A. **CORRECT:** Viral infections or certain genetic links can trigger an autoimmune response that causes type 1 diabetes mellitus.

   B. Beta cells are damaged in type 1 diabetes mellitus.

   C. **CORRECT:** Type 1 diabetes mellitus usually occurs before age 30.

   D. Type 1 diabetes mellitus is treated with insulin only.

   E. **CORRECT:** Regular exercise can reduce insulin requirements in a client who has type 1 diabetes mellitus.

   Ⓝ *NCLEX® Connection: Physiological Adaptation, Illness Management*

2. A. Fruity breath odor is a manifestation of hyperglycemia.

   B. **CORRECT:** A client who has hypoglycemia can have diaphoresis and cool, clammy skin.

   C. Ketones in the urine is a manifestation of hyperglycemia.

   D. Polyuria (excessive urination) is a manifestation of hyperglycemia.

   Ⓝ *NCLEX® Connection: Reduction of Risk Potential, System Specific Assessments*

3. A. IV insulin is administered for hyperglycemia.

   B. **CORRECT:** The client has manifestations of hypoglycemia. The nurse should offer the client 10 to 15 g of carbohydrate, such as 120 mL juice.

   C. IV potassium is administered for hypokalemia.

   D. IV sodium bicarbonate is administered for metabolic acidosis.

   Ⓝ *NCLEX® Connection: Reduction of Risk Potential, System Specific Assessments*

4. A. **CORRECT:** Carbohydrates should be 45% to 60% of total daily calorie intake.

   B. The client should avoid using hydrogenated oils for cooking because they contain trans fatty acids and increase the risk for hyperlipidemia.

   C. **CORRECT:** The client can use table sugar as long as adequate insulin or other agents are provided to cover the sugar intake.

   D. **CORRECT:** The client can drink an alcoholic beverage with meals.

   E. **CORRECT:** The client can exchange carbohydrates as long as portion size remains the same.

   Ⓝ *NCLEX® Connection: Physiological Adaptation, Illness Management*

5. A. **CORRECT:** The nurse should include weight management in the plan of care if the client is overweight.

   B. **CORRECT:** The nurse should include the client's lipid profile to determine if a plan of care is needed for hyperlipidemia.

   C. **CORRECT:** The nurse should consider the client's cultural needs when developing a plan of care for management of type 2 diabetes mellitus.

   D. A client's sleep pattern is not relevant in the dietary plan of care for a client who has type 2 diabetes mellitus.

   E. **CORRECT:** The nurse should consider the client's personal preferences regarding food and activity when developing a plan of care for management of type 2 diabetes mellitus.

   Ⓝ *NCLEX® Connection: Basic Care and Comfort, Nutrition and Oral Hydration*

PRACTICE Answer

Using the ATI Active Learning Template: System Disorder

INTERPROFESSIONAL CARE: Dietitian: Development of meal planning based on healthy food choices to meet the client's needs.

CLIENT EDUCATION
- Review of exchange list: Incorporate proteins, carbohydrates, and fats within each group based on the client's needs.
- Review of carbohydrate counting: Consider the total grams of carbohydrates in each food item and the quantity needed for each meal and snack.
- Review information on food labels: Teach how to read food labels to identify amounts of carbohydrates contained in food.

Ⓝ *NCLEX® Connection: Physiological Adaptation, Illness Management*

UNIT 3 ALTERATIONS IN NUTRITION

CHAPTER 16 *Cancer and Immunosuppression Disorders*

Nurses should be knowledgeable of nutritional needs for clients who have cancer and immunosuppression disorders. Cancer and cancer treatments can affect chewing, swallowing, satiety, digestion, taste, appetite, nutrient absorption, use of glucose, and stool formation (dependent on type).

Protein-calorie malnutrition and body wasting are common secondary diagnoses for clients who have cancer or immunosuppression disorders (HIV/AIDS). Nutritional deficits are a major cause of morbidity and mortality for these clients. Adverse effects of treatments compromise the nutritional status of affected clients. Immunosuppression disorders increase the body's nutrient demand, storage, and accessibility. They also cause a loss of lean body tissue.

The goals of nutritional therapy are to minimize the nutritional complications of disease, improve nutritional status, prevent muscle wasting, maintain weight, promote healing, reduce adverse effects, decrease morbidity and mortality, and enhance quality of life and overall effectiveness of treatment therapies. Nutritional plans are individualized for client needs.

ASSESSMENT/DATA COLLECTION

- Current illness and presence of other medical diagnoses
- Nutritional habits, food preferences, and restrictions
- Food allergies
- Height, weight, body mass index (BMI), weight trends

RISK FACTORS

Immunosuppression disorders

- Unprotected sex (HIV)
- Use of contaminated needles, such as with injection substance use (HIV)
- Use of medications that have immunosuppressive effects (cytotoxic medications, corticosteroids, disease modifying immunosuppressive medications)
- History of radiation treatment
- Congenital immune deficiencies

Cancer

- Obesity
- Sedentary lifestyle
- Consumption of processed meats, red meats, refined grains
- Excessive alcohol intake
- Family history
- History of cigarette smoking

LABORATORY TESTS

Albumin, ferritin, serum transferrin

NUTRITIONAL GUIDELINES AND NURSING INTERVENTIONS

Immunosuppression

- Instruct the client on potential food sources of bacteria (raw fruits and vegetables, undercooked meat, poultry, or eggs). Wash fruits and vegetables. Cook foods thoroughly. Refrigerate perishable foods as soon as possible. Qs
- Monitor the effectiveness of nutrition (client weight, BMI, laboratory findings).
- Teach the client to make food choices based on nutrition recommendations.
- Assist the client to set realistic goals for nutrition and food consumption.
- Instruct the client on strategies to manage adverse effects of treatment.

Cancer

Excess body fat stimulates the production of estrogen and progesterone, which can intensify the growth of various cell types and can contribute to breast, gallbladder, colon, prostate, uterine, and kidney cancers.

PREVENTATIVE NUTRITION

- Consume adequate dietary fiber (14 g per 1,000 kcal daily) to lessen the risk of colon cancer.
- Eliminate tobacco to reduce the risk of lung cancer.
- Eat at least five servings of fruits and vegetables daily (linked to a lowered incidence of many types of cancer), especially the following.
  - Foods high in vitamin A (apricots, carrots, leafy green vegetables)
  - Foods high in vitamin C (citrus fruits)
  - Cruciferous vegetables (broccoli, cauliflower, cabbage)
- Consume whole grains rather than processed or refined grains and sugars.
- Avoid meat prepared by smoking, pickling, charcoal and grilling, and use of nitrate-containing chemicals (possibly carcinogenic).
- Consume polyunsaturated and monounsaturated fats (found in fish and olive oil), which might be beneficial in lowering the risk of many types of cancer.
- Limit alcohol consumption (associated with many types of cancers).

THERAPEUTIC NUTRITION

- Cancer can cause anorexia, increased metabolism, and negative nitrogen balance.
- Systemic effects result in poor food intake, increased nutrient and energy needs, and catabolism of body tissues.
- Creating an individualized plan for the client who has cancer is based on the following. Qpcc
  - Increased caloric needs ranging from 25 to 35 cal/kg (depending on metabolism, activity level, disease state, and ability to absorb nutrients).
  - Protein needs are increased to 1.0 to 2.5 g/kg.
  - Vitamin and mineral supplementation is based upon the client's needs.

NURSING ACTIONS

- Encourage clients to eat more on days when feeling better (on "good" days).
- Encourage nutritional supplements that are high in protein and/or calories as between-meal snacks. When necessary, use as a meal replacement.
- Increase protein and caloric content of foods.
  - Substitute whole milk for water in recipes.
  - Add milk, cheese, yogurt, or ice cream to dishes.
  - Use peanut butter as a spread for fruits.
  - Use yogurt as a topping for fruit.
  - Dip meats in eggs, milk, and bread crumbs before cooking.
- Use semisolid, thickened foods for clients who have dysphagia, and instruct them to sit upright and tilt their head forward when swallowing. Qs

HIV/AIDS

THERAPEUTIC NUTRITION

- The body's response to the inflammatory and immune processes associated with HIV increases nutrient requirements. Malnutrition is common and is one cause of death in clients who have AIDS.
- HIV infection, secondary infection, malignancies, and medication therapies can cause manifestations and adverse effects that impair intake and alter metabolism.
- Creating an individualized plan for the client who has HIV/AIDS is based on the following.
  - Increased caloric needs, ranging from 37 to 55 cal/kg.
  - A high-protein diet is recommended with amounts varying from 1.2 to 2.0 g/kg/day.
  - Intake of a multivitamin that meets 100% of the recommended daily servings is sufficient, unless a specific deficiency is identified.
- Decreased nutrient intake occurs due to physical manifestations (anorexia, nausea, vomiting, diarrhea). Psychological manifestations can include depression and dementia.
- Nutritional findings include rapid weight loss, gastrointestinal problems, inadequate intake, increased nutrient needs, food aversions, fad diets, and supplements.
- Enteral feedings are used if the client is unable to consume sufficient nutrients, calories, and fluid.
- Encourage the client to consume small, frequent meals that are composed of high-protein, high-calorie, nutrient-dense foods.
- Poor nutritional status leads to wasting and fever, further increasing susceptibility to secondary infections.
- HIV-associated wasting is characterized by unintended weight loss of 10% and at least one concurrent problem (diarrhea, chronic weakness, or fever) for at least 30 days.
- Diarrhea and malabsorption are prominent clinical problems in clients who have AIDS.
- Liberal fluid intake is extremely important to prevent dehydration.

COMPLICATIONS

Early satiety and anorexia

CLIENT EDUCATION
- Eat small amounts of high-protein foods loaded with calories and nutrients.
- Try to consume food in the morning when appetite is best.
- Avoid food odors.
- Do not fill up on low-calorie foods (liquids, broth, high-roughage foods containing water).
- Eat cool or room temperature foods.

Mouth ulcers and stomatitis

CLIENT EDUCATION
- Use a soft toothbrush to clean teeth after eating and at bedtime.
- Avoid mouth washes that contain alcohol.
- Omit acidic, spicy, dry, or coarse foods.
- Include cold or room-temperature foods in the diet.
- Cut food into small bites.
- Try using straws.
- Replace meals with high-calorie/protein drinks.
- Use well-fitting dentures.

Fatigue

CLIENT EDUCATION
- Eat a large, calorie-dense breakfast when energy level is the highest.
- Conserve energy by eating foods that are easy to prepare.
- Use a meal delivery service.

Food aversions

CLIENT EDUCATION: Eat foods that are well-tolerated and liked prior to treatments (chemotherapy, radiation). Qpcc

Taste alterations and thick saliva

CLIENT EDUCATION
- Try adding foods that are tart (citrus juices).
- Eat small, frequent meals.
- Try using sauces and seasonings for added flavor.
- Use plastic utensils for eating.
- Suck on mints, candy, or chew gum to remove bad taste in mouth.

Gastrointestinal problems

CLIENT EDUCATION

Nausea, vomiting
- Eat cold or room-temperature foods.
- Try high-carbohydrate, low-fat foods.
- Avoid fried foods.
- Do not eat prior to chemotherapy or radiation.
- Take prescribed antiemetic medication.
- Sit up for 1 hr after a meal.

Diarrhea
- Ensure adequate intake of liquids throughout the day to replace losses.
- Avoid foods that can exacerbate diarrhea (foods high in roughage).
- Consume foods high in pectin to increase the bulk of the stool and to lengthen transition time in the colon.
- Limit caffeine, hot or cold drinks, and fatty foods.

Application Exercises

1. A nurse is teaching a client who has cancer about ways to increase protein and calories in foods. Which of the following actions should the nurse include? (Select all that apply.)

   A. Use peanut butter as a spread on crackers.

   B. Add water in place of milk in soups.

   C. Top fruit with yogurt.

   D. Dip chicken in eggs before cooking.

   E. Sprinkle cheese on a baked potato.

2. A nurse is teaching a community program on nutritional guidelines for cancer prevention. Which of the following instructions should the nurse include? (Select all that apply.)

   A. Eat foods high in vitamin A.

   B. Add cruciferous vegetables.

   C. Increase intake of red meats.

   D. Use saturated cooking oil.

   E. Consume refined grains.

3. A nurse in an oncology clinic is caring for a client who is undergoing treatment for cancer and reports difficulty eating due to inability to taste food. Which of the following interventions should the nurse recommend?

   A. Avoid citrus juices.

   B. Use plastic utensils to eat.

   C. Eat foods that are warm.

   D. Increase foods high in pectin.

4. A nurse is teaching a client who is undergoing cancer treatment about interventions to manage stomatitis. Which of the following statements by the client indicates understanding of the teaching?

   A. "I will try chewing larger pieces of food."

   B. "I will avoid toasting my bread."

   C. "I will consume more food in the morning."

   D. "I will add more citrus foods to my diet."

5. A nurse is collecting data from a client who has suspected HIV-associated muscle wasting. Which of the following findings supports this diagnosis?

   A. BMI 26

   B. Fecal impaction

   C. Report of fever for 30 days

   D. Report of high alcohol consumption

PRACTICE Active Learning Scenario

A nurse in an oncology clinic is reviewing dietary management with a group of clients who have cancer and are undergoing treatment. What instructions should the nurse include in this discussion? Use the ATI Active Learning Template: System Disorder to complete this item.

CLIENT EDUCATION
- Describe three effects of cancer on nutrition.
- Describe three nutritional needs.
- Describe three activities that promote improved nutrition.

1. A. **CORRECT:** Peanut butter adds calories and protein to fruit slices or crackers.

   B. The client should substitute whole milk, cream, and/or hard-boiled eggs to soups and sauces to increase protein and calories.

   C. **CORRECT:** Yogurt adds protein and calories to fruit.

   D. **CORRECT:** Eggs add protein and calories to chicken, fish, or meat.

   E. **CORRECT:** Cheese adds protein and calories to vegetables.

   Ⓝ *NCLEX® Connection: Basic Care and Comfort, Nutrition and Oral Hydration*

2. A. **CORRECT:** Consuming foods high in vitamin A, such as apricots, carrots, and leafy green vegetables, reduces the risk of cancer.

   B. **CORRECT:** Consuming cruciferous vegetables, such as broccoli and cabbage, reduces the risk the risk of cancer.

   C. Increased consumption of red meat can increase the risk for cancer.

   D. The use of polyunsaturated and monounsaturated fats is beneficial in lowering the risk of many types of cancer.

   E. Consuming whole grains reduces the risk for colon cancer.

   Ⓝ *NCLEX® Connection: Health Promotion and Maintenance, Health Promotion/Disease Prevention*

3. A. The client undergoing cancer treatment who has altered taste should try adding tart foods to the diet to increase food taste and reduce the occurrence of a metallic taste.

   B. **CORRECT:** The use of plastic utensils when eating can enhance taste sensations for the client undergoing cancer treatment and reduce the occurrence of a metallic taste.

   C. The client undergoing cancer treatment who has altered taste might find that eating cold or room-temperature foods improves taste sensation.

   D. The client undergoing cancer treatment and experiencing diarrhea should add pectin-rich foods to increase bulk of the stool and lengthen transition time in the colon.

   Ⓝ *NCLEX® Connection: Basic Care and Comfort, Nutrition and Oral Hydration*

4. A. The client should be encouraged to cut food into small pieces to reduce irritation to mucous membranes.

   B. **CORRECT:** Dry, coarse foods such as toast can worsen the manifestations of stomatitis.

   C. This intervention is indicated for the client who has fatigue due to cancer treatment.

   D. Acidic or spicy foods irritate the mucous membranes of the client who has stomatitis due to cancer treatment.

   Ⓝ *NCLEX® Connection: Basic Care and Comfort, Nutrition and Oral Hydration*

5. A. A BMI of 26 is within the expected reference range and is not a clinical finding in a client who has HIV-associated muscle wasting.

   B. A client who has HIV-associated muscle wasting will report having diarrhea, not a fecal impaction, which is found in a client who has constipation.

   C. **CORRECT:** A client who has HIV-associated muscle wasting will report elevated temperature of over 30 days duration.

   D. A client report of high alcohol consumption is not a clinical finding in HIV-associated muscle wasting.

   Ⓝ *NCLEX® Connection: Physiological Adaptation, Alterations in Body Systems*

PRACTICE Answer

Using the ATI Active Learning Template: System Disorder

CLIENT EDUCATION

Effects of cancer on nutrition
- Causes anorexia
- Increases metabolism
- Causes negative nitrogen balance

Nutritional needs
- Increased calories (25 to 35 cal/kg)
- Increased protein (1 to 2.5 g/kg)
- Vitamin and mineral supplementation

Activities
- Eat more on days when feeling better.
- Consume nutritional supplements that are high in protein and/or calories between meals and/or use as meal replacement.
- Substitute whole milk for water in recipes.
- Add milk, cheese, yogurt, or ice cream to foods when cooking.
- Add peanut butter and yogurt as a spread/topping on fruits.
- Coat meats in eggs, milk, and bread crumbs before cooking.
- Treat cancer-associated complications, such as early satiety, anorexia, mouth ulcers and stomatitis, fatigue, food aversions, altered taste, thick saliva, nausea, vomiting, and diarrhea.

Ⓝ *NCLEX® Connection: Physiological Adaptation, Illness Management*

References

Berman, A., Snyder, S., & Frandsen, G. (2016). *Kozier & Erb's fundamentals of nursing: Concepts, process, and practice* (10th ed.). Upper Saddle River, NJ: Prentice-Hall.

Burchum, J. R., & Rosenthal, L. D. (2016). *Lehne's pharmacology for nursing care* (9th ed.). St. Louis: Elsevier.

Dudek, S. G. (2014). *Nutrition essentials for nursing practice* (7th ed.). Philadelphia: Lippincott Williams & Wilkins.

Eliopoulos, C. (2014). *Gerontological nursing* (8th ed.). Philadelphia: Lippincott Williams & Wilkins.

Grodner, M., Escott-Stump, S., & Dorner, S. (2016). *Nutritional foundations and clinical applications of nutrition: A nursing approach* (6th ed.). St. Louis, MO: Mosby.

Halter, M. J. (2014). *Varcarolis' foundations of psychiatric mental health nursing: A clinical approach* (7th ed.). St. Louis, MO: Saunders.

Hockenberry, M. J., & Wilson, D. (2015) *Wong's nursing care of infants and children* (10th ed.). St. Louis, MO: Mosby.

Ignatavicius, D. D., & Workman, M. L. (2016). *Medical-surgical nursing* (8th ed.). St. Louis, MO: Elsevier.

Lowdermilk, D. L., Perry, S. E., Cashion, M. C., & Aldean, K. R. (2016). *Maternity & women's health care* (11th ed.). St. Louis, MO: Elsevier.

Pagana, K. D. & Pagana, T. J. (2014). *Mosby's manual of diagnostic and laboratory tests* (5th ed.). St. Louis, MO: Elsevier.

Pillitteri, A. (2014). *Maternal and child health nursing: Care of the childbearing and childrearing family* (7th ed.). Philadelphia: Lippincott Williams & Wilkins.

Potter, P. A., Perry, A. G., Stockert, P., & Hall, A. (2013). *Fundamentals of nursing* (8th ed.). St. Louis, MO: Mosby.

Stanhope, M., & Lancaster, J. (2014). *Foundations of nursing in the community* (4th ed.). St. Louis, MO: Mosby.

STUDENT NAME _____

CONCEPT_____ REVIEW MODULE CHAPTER_____

Related Content

(E.G., DELEGATION,
LEVELS OF PREVENTION,
ADVANCE DIRECTIVES)

Underlying Principles

Nursing Interventions

WHO? WHEN? WHY? HOW?

STUDENT NAME _____

PROCEDURE NAME _____   REVIEW MODULE CHAPTER_____

Description of Procedure

Indications

CONSIDERATIONS

Nursing Interventions (pre, intra, post)

Interpretation of Findings

Client Education

Potential Complications

Nursing Interventions

STUDENT NAME _____

DEVELOPMENTAL STAGE _____ REVIEW MODULE CHAPTER_____

EXPECTED GROWTH AND DEVELOPMENT

Physical Development	Cognitive Development	Psychosocial Development	Age-Appropriate Activities

Health Promotion

Immunizations	Health Screening	Nutrition	Injury Prevention

ACTIVE LEARNING TEMPLATE: *Medication*

STUDENT NAME _____

MEDICATION _____   REVIEW MODULE CHAPTER_____

CATEGORY CLASS_____

PURPOSE OF MEDICATION

Expected Pharmacological Action

Therapeutic Use

Complications

Medication Administration

Contraindications/Precautions

Nursing Interventions

Interactions

Client Education

Evaluation of Medication Effectiveness

STUDENT NAME _____

SKILL NAME_____ REVIEW MODULE CHAPTER_____

Description of Skill

Indications

CONSIDERATIONS

Nursing Interventions (pre, intra, post)

Outcomes/Evaluation

Client Education

Potential Complications

Nursing Interventions

STUDENT NAME _____

DISORDER/DISEASE PROCESS _____ REVIEW MODULE CHAPTER_____

Alterations in Health (Diagnosis)	Pathophysiology Related to Client Problem	Health Promotion and Disease Prevention

ASSESSMENT

Risk Factors

Expected Findings

Laboratory Tests

Diagnostic Procedures

SAFETY CONSIDERATIONS

PATIENT-CENTERED CARE

Nursing Care

Medications

Client Education

Therapeutic Procedures

Interprofessional Care

Complications

Therapeutic Procedure

STUDENT NAME _____

PROCEDURE NAME _____ REVIEW MODULE CHAPTER_____

Description of Procedure

Indications

CONSIDERATIONS

Nursing Interventions (pre, intra, post)

Outcomes/Evaluation

Client Education

Potential Complications

Nursing Interventions